NOT TONIGHT, HONEY

WHY WOMEN ACTUALLY DON'T WANT SEX AND WHAT WE CAN DO ABOUT IT

COURTNEY BOYER

ISBN: 979-8-218-19522-9

Any references to historical events, real people, or real places are used fictitiously. Names, characters, and places are products of the author's imagination.

Book cover design by iDea Signs

Author picture by Liz Webster

First printing edition 2023.

WORKBOOK LINK

To get the most of your reading experience, download the free
Workbook by going to
www.courtneyboyercoaching.com/workbook

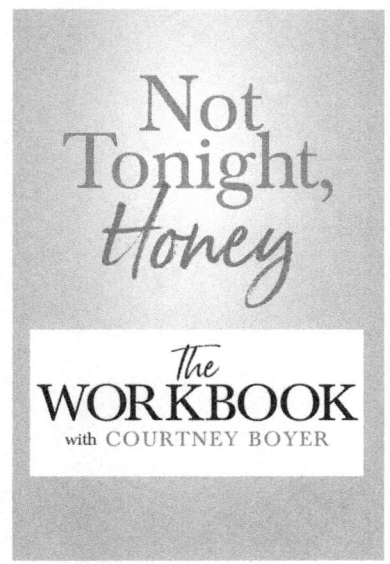

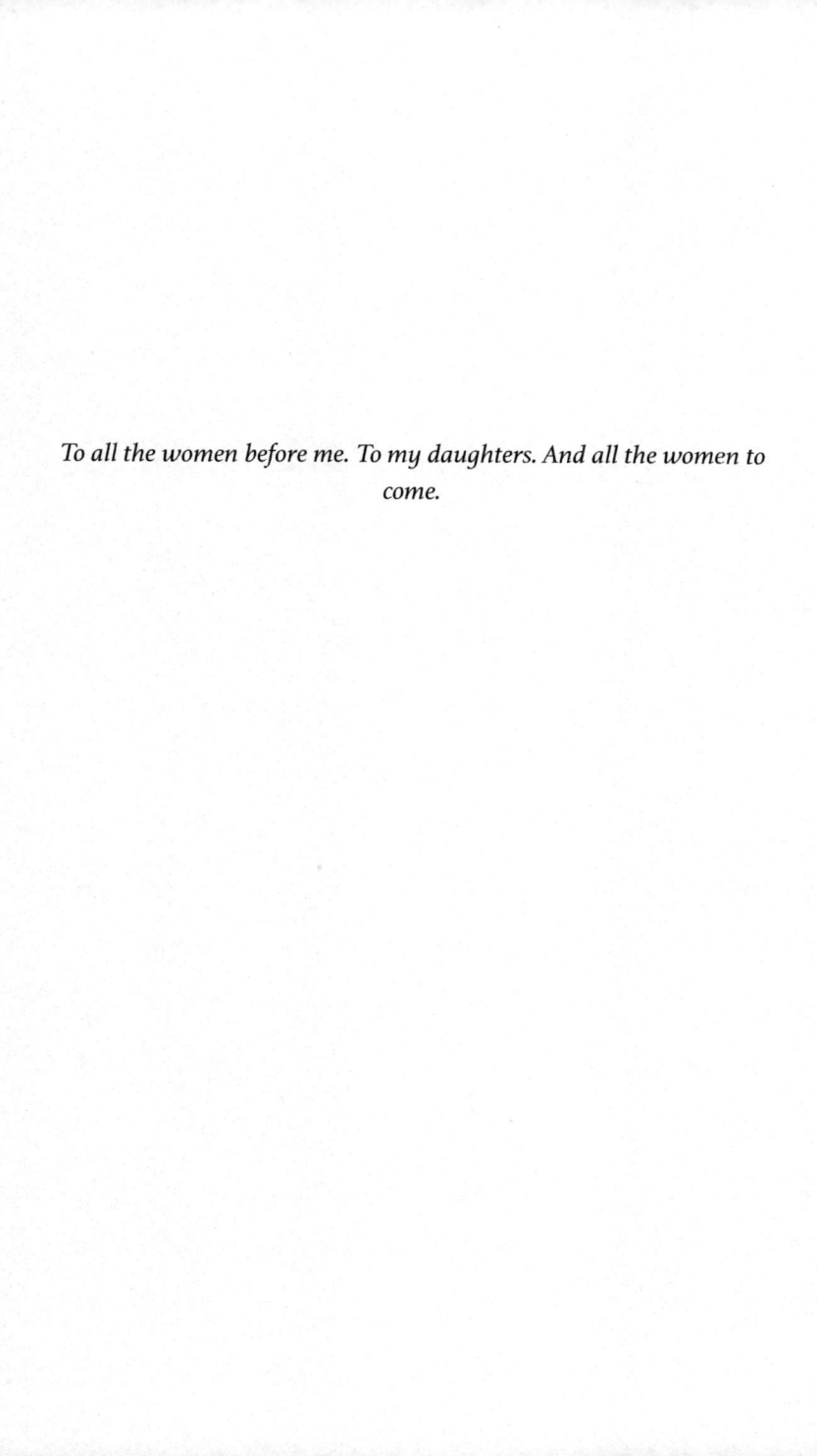

To all the women before me. To my daughters. And all the women to come.

INTRODUCTION

"I'm not really interested in anything anymore," Shanae told me. "My days are spent taking care of my kids, taking care of my spouse, going to work, and coming home. I put everyone's needs before my own and I have no energy left."

"What do you like to do for fun?" I asked her.

She laughed and paused, "Oh, you're serious? Well, I um, I don't have time for fun."

I nodded my head and asked her, "Ok, so, if you could create a day of fun for yourself, what would that look like?"

She crossed her arms and leaned back in her chair. "Hmm... I, well..." she began. A minute went by, and she began to smile. "I'd drive myself to the beach and paint," she finally said.

"Oh that sounds great," I said. "I want you to be more specific though. How would you drive to the beach? In silence?"

She shook her head, "Hell no. I'd crank that gangsta rap all the way up," she said as she began to laugh.

In just those few minutes, Shanae began to come alive.

For a multitude of reasons, Shanae's sexual energy was blocked. She felt stuck in the monotony of her daily routine. She had no interest in sex because she had a hard time seeing herself as anything more than a working mom who was also a maid and chauffeur. Shanae's mood was pretty flat most of the time. She lacked warmth and often came across as a bit rigid. Shanae struggled in finding pleasure in most things. Everything felt like a task, a chore, with a few moments here and there of love and tenderness.

Shanae was going through life to check the boxes. Kids fed and off to school? Check. Off to work? Check. Groceries bought? Check. Meals made? Check. Church on Sunday? Check. Sex with partner? Check. Call Mom? Check.

It's not that having a to-do list is bad—not at all. It's when our *lives* become the to-do list that it becomes problematic. If you like to write lists, consider the last time you put something FUN on there. Dance party? Painting? Gardening? Scrapbooking? Solo trip? (And I don't mean going to Target by yourself.) And it doesn't count if those activities were really ulterior ways to burn calories, further your education, get volunteer hours, or do something for your business. Because when we do this, we're missing the point. I know I was.

And that's what I see so many women doing. We're missing the point of this life. I used to see life as one big accomplishment with specific milestones that needed to be achieved along the way. Married by 22? Check. Kids by 30? Check. Successful spouse? Check. Homeowner? Check. Check. Check.

I was burning myself out to get those boxes checked. And when I was on the verge of breaking down, I asked myself, what am I doing all this for? Who am I really doing this for? Is any of this actually making me happy?

Sadly, we're making this life about doing and achieving, and all the while we're missing out on just *being*. Being ourselves. Being present. Being loved. Being free. We are letting the joy of this life get sucked out of us for the sake of "success."

And let me tell you, I have worked with some incredibly successful people: doctors, lawyers, engineers, professors, entrepreneurs. These individuals have gorgeous families, beautiful homes, and country club memberships. They spend time at church on Sunday and send their kids to great schools. They work hard! And despite all of that, most of them are miserable. Not all the time, but there's a deep current running through them that threatens to swallow them up some days.

Even outwardly successful people refuse to acknowledge this threat because they don't believe they have the time or the energy to deal with it. They're scared that maybe everything they've worked for, everything they've achieved, isn't the ultimate answer to happiness and fulfillment. And they have no idea what truly inspires them because they're too busy pushing through.

What if the answer, or even part of it, lies within us? What if we could find out what inspires us? What brings us passion? What makes us feel alive? And in turn, we became examples for others. For our children.

But most importantly, what if we honor ourselves?

What if we connected with the life force inside of us?

What if we learned to honor our mind, body, and spirit?

What if we embraced our desires?

What if we welcomed our emotions?

What if we celebrated our feminine power?

What if we gave ourselves permission to be the sexual beings we are?

Maybe, just maybe, we could change the world.

What This Book is About

You may be thinking, I thought this book was about how to have more sex. Isn't this supposed to help me fix my low (or lost) desire for sex problem? Yes, this book is about sex, and I promise, there will be plenty of tips for increasing your libido. But what I have found is that the reason many women struggle with their desire for sex is not because they are refusing to try.

I'm sure you've tried very hard for many years. You've scoured the local bookshelves and blogs for answers. For anything, really, that would increase your interest in sex. A tip (or 12) that would help you meet your partner's sexual requests (or demands). Something that finally explains what's "wrong" with you. I get it. I've been there.

And so have countless women before you. This book isn't just a factual read through. It's filled with clinical vignettes (either compilations of actual client sessions or specific client situations, always used with permission), anecdotes, and exercises all inspired by the latest research.

I didn't want to write a stuffy book citing scientific studies. I wanted a guidebook where women could see themselves reflected in the pages. Where they felt validated and seen. A book that would enable them to walk away with realistic action steps so they could start creating the life they once dreamed of. I want that so badly for you. I remember what it was like to feel defeated and discouraged, and I'm here to tell you that it can be different. It truly can.

My Journey

"How do you want to feel?" my life coach asked me during our session.

"Powerful," I immediately responded.

"Why?" she asked.

For someone who thinks quickly and usually has an answer ready, I couldn't find one to give her. I avoided giving the standard, "I dunno," answer I often get from my own clients when they haven't done the work to really ascertain why.

"Um," I slowly began, biding my time. "I guess 'cause it feels good. I want to feel powerful because then I'm in charge and I don't have to rely on others," I blurted out, hoping that response would suffice. We moved on to something else, but I continued thinking about this conversation.

The truth is, I didn't really know at the time WHY I wanted to feel this way. I could feel the energy in my solar plexus (the chakra associated with our self-worth and self-image) surge when I gave that answer, but it didn't feel complete.

A few months later, I was in the shower (where so many great discoveries have been made) and I finally realized why I desired power. Feeling powerful was something I never possessed. For my entire life, I had always been at the whim of someone else's rules, norms, or expectations. I was the product of the evangelical system, a mainstream religious organization that permeates American culture, education, and politics. Despite being a people pleaser, I could never get myself to fit the mold of the meek and mild Christian woman.

I was intelligent, outspoken, attractive, assertive, athletic, and contemplative. If I were a man, I would have been celebrated. But as a woman, I was told I was too much. Too bossy, too loud, too disagreeable, too distracting, and too sexual. The message I internalized wasn't that I was "too much."

Instead, I began to believe that it wasn't safe to be in my body. That I took up too much space physically, sexually, emotionally, and spiritually. And when you do not feel safe in your body, you learn how to hide from yourself. It's incredibly difficult to be present in life, let alone engage in a sexual encounter, when you are looking for ways to escape.

So I did. I escaped into the pursuit of success. And boy did I check all the boxes. By the time I was 30 years old, I was happily married to a physician in the military (who was about to start a competitive fellowship); had three healthy, beautiful children; completed two master's degrees; owned several businesses; bought three homes; taught at a university; and had a thriving private practice.

Here's the thing: no matter what I did, it was never enough. I consistently pushed myself to be better. Smarter. Thinner. Stronger. Prettier. I hated my body for not being what I thought it should be, feeling betrayed anytime I walked by a mirror and it reflected back a woman who just couldn't get it "right."

You know what that led to? Burnout. Disordered Eating. Resentment. Frustration. Anxiety. Depression.

It also led to loneliness. When you're trying to prove that you deserve a seat at the table, you isolate and withdraw from others. Sure, I had lots of acquaintances and friends. And I was really good at putting on a front to convince them that everything was great.

All the while, I was desperately seeking approval and accolades from others. And boy, was I good at getting them. The applause. The admiration. But it never filled me up for very long. I found myself chasing that high. That Supermom status. Becoming a slave to a life I wasn't even happy with.

So I set out searching for something new. Determined to find joy. Despite being a clinically trained mental health and sex therapist, I didn't feel like I had the right tools. Traditional talk therapy wasn't working for me. Something was missing. There had to be more.

Eventually, I discovered coaching. As a military spouse, this field aligned perfectly with our lifestyle of moving every few years since unlike therapy, licensure is not required. I decided to pursue a coaching certification. After I completed it in 2018, I began to realize how destructive my beliefs and thought processes were. But more importantly, I realized that I had the power to change them.

But something still felt like it was missing. So I continued exploring both personally and professionally. In early 2021, I began to understand the pervasive disconnection between mind and body and wanted to learn more about healing this chasm. I became a certified level 2 reiki practitioner to help clients integrate and reconcile their minds and bodies. I continue to train in different modalities, adding powerful tools to my toolbox to help others. That thirst for knowledge has never stopped, but it's no longer fueled by feelings of inadequacy.

It's incredible, given the number of accomplished women I've worked with, to see how pervasive their sense of inadequacy is, especially sexually. There's a belief that if we consume enough knowledge and make it to the top of that mountain, we'll finally have it all figured out. Spoiler alert—I'm a highly educated relationship and sexuality expert, and I still don't have things figured out. But I've finally realized, that's not my job. My job, which is one of the great privileges I have in this life, is to guide those who feel they've lost their way. Who are wandering aimlessly, believing they are broken or unwanted, wondering if they belong. Disappointed, discontented, disconnected, and depleted. Those are my people.

If that resonates with you, if you feel like you're among those

I just described, I want you to know how grateful I am that you are reading these words. My life's work is about educating, equipping, and empowering others to live authentically free lives. I hope this book will help you on your journey to reclaiming that sacred part of yourself.

Before we begin, I want you to consider a few things. It may be helpful for you to grab a pen and notebook or open the notes app on your phone. Or if you haven't already, download the free workbook from my website. These questions will impact the way you receive these pages.

- Why did you pick up this book?
- Who are you reading this for?
- Why are you doing this? Why are you investing your time, money, and energy into reading this book?

There's no wrong answers to these questions. And you could honestly just breeze right on by them. But I think it's important to acknowledge your intention before you begin.

It's something I asked myself every time I sat down at my computer to write—what do I hope my reader learns? What am I trying to convey? Who am I doing this for? Answering those questions kept me centered. Kept me focused on finishing. Kept me tethered to the belief that one person can make a difference. I hope that however you answer those questions, you feel encouraged. Hopeful. Curious.

PART I

HOW DID WE GET HERE?

I'm a big fan of metaphors. I want you to imagine a gorgeous lake standing before you. When I picture it, I see mountains surrounding a teal blue pool of water. As I imagine this serene scene, a sense of calm comes over me. As you picture your own body of water before you, I want you to get right up to the water line. This is a time when we don't just put our toes in the water. No, ma'am. We are gonna wade all the way in. We will take in our surroundings and as we do, witness the ripples around us. Not just the ripples that we created, but also the ripples of our fellow sisters. Because you are not alone in this water. You are surrounded. Supported.

The women in the water with you, as you will see throughout this book, face the same challenges you do. And yet, we are often made to feel alone in these struggles. Look around and see. See that we are all connected. As women, we belong to a special sisterhood. Even if most days, it doesn't really feel that way.

(It's important for me to note that I use the word *woman* to describe anyone who identifies as one. If that's you, then this book is for you.)

Let's start by taking a comprehensive look at where we have been as women and as a society. I wanted to answer the questions, "How did we get here?" How did we get to a place where we need a book for women who struggle to desire sex? These first chapters are a journey through our collective history and the contemporary messaging on sexuality, relationships, and the role of religion. It's a hard look at our past that I believe is necessary because it allows us to face our future more authentically.

As we consider where we've been, it requires us to take a look in the mirror. And I mean that literally. Despite being one of the simplest activities, mirror work is one of my favorite exercises (we'll cover that later) because it's powerful. It feels odd. And it's uncomfortable because it requires vulnerability many of us are not used to. Which is exactly why it's the work we need to help us take stock and consider where we want to go.

So buckle up, sister, because it's going to be a bit of a bumpy ride.

ALL THE REASONS WHY

I sat cross legged on the hard gym floor, fixated on the pretty blonde coach speaking to me and hundreds of other female athletes there for my junior high summer basketball camp. "When you go back to your room tonight, I want you to pull out your notebook and write your future husband a letter," the speaker instructed us.

Idealistic and obedient, I went back to my dorm room, sat at the wooden desk, and began writing to a man I was told would love and honor me forever. My 14-year-old hand excitedly gushed out love and devotion to the future man of my dreams on those pages.

The next night, we came back, letters in hand. The pretty blonde woman continued, "imagine giving this letter to him on your wedding night... Do you think he'd want to know that he's shared you [sexually] with other people? Doesn't he deserve a wife who's preserved her purity and saved herself only for him?"

A sea of heads nodded in agreement with the speaker. We were transfixed, blankly staring at the woman speaking passionately about sexual abstinence: "Isn't your future marriage, your future family, worth waiting for?"

This was a common message girls like me received growing up in the Evangelical Christian Church. One of the messages preached to us consistently was that you cannot give this part of yourself (your virtue, your heart, your soul, your body) away to someone unless you were married. Sex before marriage wasn't just sinful; it was shameful.

I remember during a "special" school assembly, the family life educator (because there was no sex education at my Christian high school), took a single sheet of paper in hand and said, "when you have sex with someone who isn't your husband or wife, you give a piece of your heart away." Then she ripped part of the paper. "When you engage in activities in the danger zone (she referenced the diagram of what was considered safe sexual activity), you lose a little part of yourself." Rip. "The more partners you have..." Rip. "The less of you there is to give to the person you're supposed to love the most." Rip. This continued for several minutes. Finally, the speaker looked at the pieces of torn paper on the ground and then at the one small shred remaining in her hand. Message received.

So how did young, hormonal humans deal with such a decree? We disconnected from our bodies. We ignored and suppressed those sexual desires because we knew that they would ultimately betray us, and we often heard, "You cannot trust your body; it will lead you astray." The Bible verse Matthew 5:30 would frequently be cited, "And if your right hand causes you to stumble, cut it off and throw it away. It is better for you to lose one part of your body than for your whole body to go into hell" (NIV).

But what happens when your whole body feels like it's causing you to stumble? Not only do you disconnect from it; you shame it. You become disgusted with the very flesh and bones your mind and soul call home.

And you're reminded that others are also disgusted with the

most intimate parts of you. During my teen years, I remember hearing guys making taco and fish jokes about a woman's vagina. I even knew of a male restaurateur who opened a chain of restaurants controversially named, the Pink Taco, which is a slang term for a woman's vagina. My high school guy friends would talk about how some chick was too bushy or how hot it was that she shaved her pubic hair.

I'd hear the same messages in music, specifically in rap and hip-hop. Women were accessories, but more explicitly, commodities—especially women of color, whose bodies were up for appraisal. This genre merely reflected the overall misogynistic culture, promoting the prescribed gender roles to a good beat. In mainstream movies marketed to teens, women were typically portrayed as tools for sexual possession, pleasure, and domination (looking at you, *American Pie* series).

Research shows that exposure to these messages contributes to sexual harassment, objectification, and violence because it influences how men perceive women and sex. It also models for women what we believe other women think and feel about sex.

As adolescent women, we were also dealing with the new realities of our menstrual cycles. Most women of my generation felt shame, confusion, or fear when they started their period. Why? Because their mothers never taught them what to expect. Once again, no one was discussing healthy, normal developments. If they were, it was usually to associate our moodiness with PMS or dismiss us for being too emotional because we menstruate each month.

This is something I still see reflected in some of my female clients. They are quick to blame their fluctuating hormones for snapping at their kids or yelling at their spouse. Women have accepted the belief that the Red Curse is, in fact, just that.

All of this contributed to my belief that men weren't interested in understanding my body. Furthermore, an undercurrent flowed through all this that boys were just built differently. Men and women were not the same. Women were smaller and needed protecting. From what, I always wondered? Apparently, men. Because naturally, they are more sexual creatures. They NEED sex. And because of this, they are easily tempted and will buckle at the first sign of a bra strap.

Mistrust and temptation of the other sex permeate the landscape from adolescence well into adulthood. We then carry this messaging into our adult relationships. Women are raised to be wary of men because of their supposed insatiable need for sex. We were segregated in church and discouraged from having heterosexual friendships. Another aspect of ourselves that must be controlled and regulated.

Sexual Gatekeeper Syndrome

So of course, what do good Christian girls do? We take on the task of preventing our brothers in Christ from stumbling sexually. This meant we had to wear longer shorts or T-shirts instead of tank tops. We wore one-piece suits while the boys could wear swim trunks without a shirt.

I distinctly remember multiple occasions where my girlfriends were pulled out of class and sent to the office to have the length of their shorts measured by the secretary. If they were found in violation of dress code policy (shorts could not be shorter than three inches above the knee), they had to immediately change or call their parents to have them bring "appropriate clothing," all the while missing time in class. This never happened to me personally because I never wore shorts to school. I didn't think I had a good enough body shape to wear shorts, so I opted out of them.

Of course my girlfriends complained, but only to each other. We learned that appealing to the administration did no good.

Instead, we learned to suck it up, suppress our desires and take on the responsibilities of other people's actions. This belief, that we were responsible for how other people behaved, fueled the message that boys will be boys and that they just can't help their desires.

This belief was reinforced anytime someone asked of the sexual assault survivor, "but what was she wearing?" This belief was demonstrated anytime we were told, "geez, can't you take a joke" when we didn't laugh at an unwanted sexual advance or innuendo. Thankfully, we women CAN control ourselves (I mean do women even really like sex?) so make sure you hold the line, or well, your belt, so nothing's gettin' in there.

This, my sisters, is how the Sexual Gatekeeper Syndrome is born in each one of us. It's millions of micro-messages sent throughout our lives to convince us that sex is something to be regulated and resisted. Not something that was created to be enjoyed and experienced.

And because of this, we've spent our entire lives being the sexual gatekeepers of society. Yet, our male partners never understand why we don't seem to desire sex very often. Why we are the ones that always "say no." I've spoken at countless mom groups around the world, and every time I can guarantee I'll be asked this question, "how can I want sex more?" The stories I hear from these exhausted and overwhelmed mamas revolve around negotiating sex with their spouses: "My husband and I always fight about it and I just don't understand why I can't get in the mood. I'd be fine without sex, but I know he can't go without it. What can I do?"

I always smile and look the woman in the eyes because I want her to know that she is not alone. I want this woman to know that her story is the same as millions before her and many in that very room. I want her to know that it took courage to ask a question that she's been desperate for an answer to. And then I tell her this:

One reason we don't want sex goes back to being slut-shamed and called *whore* when we've said "yes" too soon or too often. We are taught that our needs don't matter as long as we've got kids and a husband who love us. We are told tales of how women's sensuality brought down entire civilizations.

We learn that our "no's" are always up for negotiation. That choosing abstinence makes us prude. So we shrink ourselves and believe the lies that we're not nearly enough. We drown our desires in food and alcohol and compulsive shopping. We focus on ways to find fulfillment, but it never feels like we've done enough. We seek solace in the stories of other women who feel just as sexually broken and inadequate as we do. As women, our sexuality isn't celebrated; it's silenced throughout our entire lives.

I let that sink in and then with a straight face I state, "I'm here to say, no more."

The Best of Intentions

It's important for me to acknowledge that I believe wholeheartedly that my parents, family, church, and school were doing their best. It's easy to look back now and think awful things about the people in our lives who imparted (mis)information to us at such a critical time in our development.

Honestly, I don't believe that anyone harbored malicious intent in their messaging even though so much of the information we received was steeped in fear. And to be fair, there was good reason. Pregnancy rates among teens had risen during the mid-1980s and peaked in 1991. The HIV/AIDS epidemic hit in the early 1980s. Within 10 years, the number one cause of death for American men between the ages of 25 and 44 was AIDS. I remember being afraid to go to the movies for a while because of the rumor that someone was putting HIV-infected needles into the seat cushions. Loads of chaotic (and medically inaccurate) information spread like wildfire, mostly about things we didn't fully understand at the time. And what we don't understand, we fear.

I don't fault those thought-leaders for their fear. However, that doesn't mean there aren't ramifications for how they acted (out of their fear), because there are and were. Creating accountability allows us to acknowledge the pain that others have caused while working toward our own healing. It's not about blame or finger-pointing. It's about understanding why we're here, struggling to connect with our bodies to enjoy sex. But I firmly believe accountability is best offered with compassion, for ourselves and for those who have hurt us, and on a very real level, still hurt us.

I talk to so many women who still hear a small voice inside them, telling them that "sex is bad" or "dirty" or "sinful." And as much as they've tried to move on and silence this shame, they don't know how to get this voice to shut up.

But seeking protection from this voice, the messaging and the institutions still associated with them can feel scary. And our brain doesn't like scary. So we settle. We perpetuate a cycle for security's sake because security is what our brain craves (at the most basic level of our human need, think Maslow's pyramid; security equals safety, and safety equals staying alive). For so many of the women in the generations before us, conforming to the role of the God-fearing, stay-at-home mother allowed them to feel safe. And what is safe? Safe is predictable and known. It's not sexy; it's not exciting. It's stable.

All the Pressure

The pressure to conform is something biologically ingrained in us. Humans are social creatures and have, for as long as we've walked this earth, survived by living in tribes and communities. That primitive part of our brain has not caught up with the fact that we can live outside a community in today's society (yes, we still need a social community, but communities are so much more fluid than they were even 50 years ago). Historically, belonging to a community meant conformity, playing by the rules set forth by the elders or politicians or leaders.

But what happens when the true essence of who you are can't conform to the standards or expectations of your community?

I spoke with Kamil, a lesbian, about her experience growing up in the Evangelical Christian Church. I asked her whether she felt there was a pressure to conform and whether she felt there were consequences for being "different":

> I didn't realize there were true life-and-death type conse-
> quences until I got to college. I also didn't realize the amount of
> self-hatred I had begun planting based on responses to indirect
> questions I'd asked of my parents and church family mentors.
> The pressure to conform was HUGE...I'd say I saw [the] conse-
> quences of being different, yes. I didn't realize that my motiva-
> tions were rooted in my attractions to the same gender until I
> got quite a bit older... I can recall conversations with my dad
> somewhere between the ages of 11 to 14 around homosexuality
> and basically coming to the conclusion that gay equals bad.
>
> So when I finally came out to him and my stepmom they
> asked, "Why did you never talk to us about this?"
>
> Well, why would I? You're the ones that have been telling
> me that being homosexual is bad and being sexually active is

bad and that masturbating is bad and handing me books by Dr. [James] Dobson to pressure me into straight purity culture. Not only that... but I couldn't admit my own homosexuality to myself at that age, let alone talk with anyone about it.

Kamil tried to hold on to what was expected of her (growing up and marrying a man) despite her attraction to women. As a child, she was forced to choose between attachment (acceptance from her family) and authenticity (being true to who she believed she was created to be).

Kamil didn't feel safe enough in her own family to explore her sexual attraction or feelings of being different as a child. So she pushed those desires into the closet to press on. In order to stay alive mentally, spiritually, and relationally. When Kamil came out as lesbian to her parents, there was push-back. Her parents gathered their defense primarily based on spiritual principles. But I see this elsewhere when young women "come out" in different ways.

Growing up, I always wanted to be a lawyer. More importantly, my dad always wanted me to be a lawyer. I fully embraced the hard work and achievements required to get me into law school until, one semester into college, I realized this wasn't actually my dream; it was my dad's.

I decided to wait to tell my dad, who was paying for my undergraduate education, until I saw him in person. A few weeks later, after driving the 4 ½ hours from one side of Washington state to the other, I sat down with my dad in our living room. "Dad, I need to tell you something," I said with tears streaming down my face. "This is really hard for me and I don't know where to start. I don't want to go to law school. I'm sorry." He could see my anguish, but in a very practical tone, he asked, "So what's your plan?" I hadn't anticipated that question, but I could sense his disappointment. Looking back, I believe he was afraid of me settling, of accepting a life that felt good enough instead of creating one that was great.

The ironic thing is that I agree with him. I don't want "good enough!" I want more. And by more I don't mean more clothes or more titles or a bigger house. There's nothing wrong with those things if that's what you truly desire. I believe we all deserve more. When you have the freedom to cultivate your desires, your happiness in life, and speak your truth, it allows you to passionately contribute to the world. When we do this, we show up as the energetic best version of ourselves.

I find this approach, living authentically, a lot better than the white-knuckling bitter survival that burns us out. As I tell my clients, there is no rule book, no guidebook telling us what we can and can't have or who we're allowed to be or love.

When we show up as our authentic, energetic selves, we are more in tune with our gifts and passions, allowing us to contribute from a place of love, rather than from insecurity and fear.

An authentic, passionate woman, rooted in love, believes she is worthy of pleasure. She is in touch with her body, connected with her body. She can feel the joy and excitement of life in every cell of her body (much like an orgasm). Not all the time, but she knows that she has that ability to tune in and draw from that energy, that never-ending well, whenever she needs to.

Whenever she wants to.

Toolbox:

- What messages did I receive as a young girl about sex, sexuality, and marriage? How have those impacted me? How do they still impact me?
- How have I chosen safety and security over my desires?
- What am I afraid of when it comes to sex, sexuality, desire, and pleasure?

2

A HISTORY OF WOMEN AND SEX

It's 1995, and I am 12 years old, watching Michael Jordan come out of his retirement to play once again as a Chicago Bull. My mom has some friends over and as any tween will do, I eavesdrop on their conversation.

"Did you hear that Brad and Maggie are moving in together?" I heard my mom's friend say to her.

"They're not even married," my mother confirmed in a hushed tone.

The conversation was quickly over, but the message had been received. I could see the looks of disdain and disapproval on their faces. I would sense the absence of these friends at parties. I would hear their names spoken differently in discussions. And I decided that I never wanted that to happen to me.

IN MY SHORT time here on Earth, I have seen the pendulum swing from the chastisement of unmarried couples living together before marriage (aka "living in sin") to the approval of individuals in open and even group marriages. And while I find this shift fascinating, I'm more interested in the centuries of female sexual behavior that led to what I have seen in my lifetime.

Why does this matter? Because those stories, those experiences of the many women before us, still run in our veins. Sometimes this is referred to as *generational trauma*. Generational trauma is the belief that big "T" (experiencing war/famine, abuse) and little "t" (divorce, moving frequently, bullying) traumatic experiences can be passed down from one generation to the next. In some religious circles, these are referred to as *generational curses*. For example, a daughter is abused by her mother and that mother was abused by her mother and so on. The growing field of epigenetics, the study of how environment and behavior can affect the way our genes work, is just starting to put the pieces of passed-down experiences together.

You may not care what Mildred's views and thoughts on sex were three hundred years ago. But that history, her history, and the history of our sisters and mothers and grandmothers before us are part of our collective story—one that cannot be easily ignored, for it has shaped our own beliefs and behaviors.

Recognizing the role these narratives have played (and continue to play) is a crucial step to beginning the healing journey, one that honors those before us and prepares a place for those to come.

Before I began my research on this subject, I honestly expected the stories to be pretty much the same: two thousand plus years of women (those of "character" or noble status) deemed as nonsexual creatures who only engaged in sex to procreate. And of course, this contrasted with the "whores" who used sex to manipulate men for money, control, or a seat at the table.

What I found actually surprised me, so much so that I found myself inspired by the stories of these women who dared to claim what was theirs. Their bodies, their femininity, their sexual prowess—they weren't always repressed. But, as I tell my children, history is told by the winners, those who find themselves in positions of power, who get to dictate the narrative. And who controls the narrative has great influence on how their citizens show up and behave.

One of the great contributors to sexual behavior throughout the centuries was medical advice. During medieval times, it was (incorrectly) believed that women needed to orgasm to conceive. This resulted in an emphasis on the female orgasm, causing husbands to be diligent in bringing their wives to climax. Sadly, this didn't last for too long.

During the Victorian era, it was believed that married couples should only have sex once a month so the woman's internal organs could recover from the exertion of such activity. Additionally, the missionary position was promoted as the gold standard for conceiving. Sex with knees drawn in or in an upright position was not recommended because these positions were believed to be a cause of cancer.

Although I don't doubt that the medical professionals of the past had good intentions, they unknowingly affected the behavior of millions of couples. But the medical profession wasn't the only voice in the ears of our foremothers.

The Church was also vying for influence. Homosexuality, masturbation, oral sex, and anal sex were all considered sinful. Pleasure was seen as a desire of the flesh, something that corrupted men and disrupted society. Sexual activity within marriage was allowed but only for procreative purposes. Contraception was banned because it allowed couples to have sex for the purpose of pleasure. Sex became an activity loaded with danger and fear, regulated by authority.

This began to create an opportunity for the Church not just to influence, but also to control society's behavior. More importantly, it taught individuals to seek answers from authority instead of reflecting within themselves. This was never promoted as an option for women.

Women were never allowed to think or act beyond their prescribed societal roles. In fact, this has been the dominant belief in many sects of Christianity. Based on one interpretation of 1 Corinthians 11:3, it is believed that the hierarchy and authority of God is ordered as follows: God the Father, Christ, the man or husband, and the woman or wife.

This hierarchy never sat well with me—not because I, as a woman, was at the bottom. But because it didn't speak to the Christ I knew who transcended gender, class, and sexual roles. Who came to set the captives free. Who sat with and loved the outcasts of his day. Who showed what Love incarnate is and does. Who accepts me exactly as I am and inspires me to be a better person.

In the early days of the Church, it was expected for Corinthian (modern day Greece) women to wear a head covering or veil; this demonstrated a woman was married, and under the authority of her husband. It's important to know that the Greco-Roman Empire declared it illegal for female slaves and prostitutes to cover their head or wear a veil. So, when married women were out in the markets, their veil-wearing meant that you couldn't rape them without consequence (because they belonged to another man).

Slaves and prostitutes were not given this protection, so they were forbidden from wearing veils. Instead, these women were sexual property, and therefore could be sexually assaulted legally; however, a married woman was considered protected. Sexually assaulting a married woman was seen as performing an offense against her husband.

The idea that women are men's property is nothing new. If you go back a few thousand years to the days of Moses and examine the sixth commandment, "You shall not commit adultery," you will find that the definition of adultery is not what we think of it today (one spouse cheating on the other spouse). Adultery was defined as having sex with another man's wife without the husband's permission. If a man offered his wife sexually to a friend or stranger, that was not considered adultery because the man had the husband's approval. Of course, the wife's opinion was irrelevant.

Getting back to Paul's writings in 1 Corinthians, this is where I find beauty in this Bible passage. Paul is telling all the women, who would have included married women and prostitutes, in his community to cover their heads. He is encouraging them to break the law because he wants the lower-class women to recover their honor and dignity by covering their heads—which, of course, implies that men should conduct themselves as if ALL women were married (protected). This is based on the belief that everyone is welcome and honored in God's community; Paul is reminding them that there is no social, gender, or class delineation in Christ.

Paul is using his position of privilege to empower these women. And yet, most Christians, specifically conservative and fundamental Christians, are unaware of the historical and cultural significance of these words in 1 Corinthians 11:2–16. I know I was; I was never taught any of this and only found the information when I went searching for it.

As much as I would love to continue examining significant chunks of church and world history, I want to continue our journey by fast-forwarding to the Puritan era. Surprisingly, many "ordinary" (non-noble) individuals included sex as part of serious courtship in the 1600s to mid-1800s. In fact, many Americans held the belief that one's health could be harmed by abstinence.

Records from the late 17th to late 18th century showed that approximately 25% of brides in certain rural areas were already pregnant on their wedding day. This number increased to nearly 40% by the end of the 19th century. Premarital sex was widely accepted for most in the working class and middle class. In fact, it only became a shameful act when the woman was left with an illegitimate child.

However, as society entered the Victorian era, premarital chastity was expected from women in the upper-middle class and upper class. Their family's reputations were at stake, after all. Marriages, while arranged like the lower classes, involved significant wealth, status, and power. Any indiscretions could threaten a powerful alliance.

This resulted in infrequent or cautious premarital relations, with many upper-class women rejecting premarital sex as unrespectable. At the same time, messages to men focused on avoiding the animalistic nature of sex and being wary of carnal passions. Could this messaging have clouded men's judgment in believing that women didn't actually enjoy sex? Possibly.

The importance of one's image changed during the Victorian Era, when a woman was seen as a direct reflection of her husband's worth. As this class of women became focused on creating the picture-perfect home, they began to see sex as beneath their proper roles as wife and mother. Sex was seen as necessary for procreation, but not something to be enjoyed, let alone discussed in polite society.

So what happens when a man's wife is taught to disregard sex, to dismiss her husband's passionate preludes? He gets his needs met elsewhere. In 1867, Alice Christina Abbott was a 17-year-old girl who was accused of poisoning her stepfather. Alice claimed that her stepfather had an "improper connection" with her since she was 13 years old. Allegedly, Alice had had enough of the abuse and threatened to tell others about his behavior. Alice's stepfather threatened to put her in a reform school if she went public. So, the story goes, Alice killed him by poisoning his tea one afternoon. Alice was ultimately sentenced to an insane asylum and was treated as a deranged individual by the media of her day.

The idea that Alice was the victim of a sex crime wasn't even in the public consciousness. How could a man commit a crime against something he owned? Women were locked away for trying to protect themselves or for having desires for something deeper than a despondent existence. The message "your body does not belong to you" continued to ring true.

In the early 1900s, the principle of "passionlessness" (lack of sexual desire) was considered typical for women. Women who deviated from this principle would have enjoyed sex, mastur-bated, or even initiated sex. In addition, any kind of assertive or litigious behavior would have been characterized as hysterical by the medical profession. One physician claimed that women suffering from "excessive" vaginal lubrication (a normal physio-logical reaction signifying arousal) were suffering from hysteria. A healthy female sexual response was now classified as a medical condition.

Husbands and fathers would hire psychiatrists to investigate the "abnormal" behaviors of their wives and daughters. What was considered abnormal at the turn of the 19th century? Overe-ducation, exhaustion, mood swings related to a woman's menstrual cycle, masturbation, just to name a few. These men would use the pretense of medicine to exert control over the lives and bodies of the women in their lives. What happened to these women? Oftentimes, they suffered the same fate as Eliza-beth Packard.

Elizabeth Packard was the wife of a conservative Calvinist pastor. At some point in their marriage, Elizabeth began to disagree with her husband's beliefs. One Sunday morning, Eliz-abeth couldn't take it anymore. She stood up in the middle of her husband's sermon and announced that she was going across the street to the Methodist church. She gathered her things and did just that.

Later that week, Elizabeth's husband, Theophilus, arranged for a doctor to visit her at their home. Theophilus knew Elizabeth wouldn't speak to a doctor, so he asked the doctor to pretend to be a sewing machine salesman. Elizabeth, ignorant of the ruse, confided in the man that she was concerned with her husband's extreme beliefs and affirmed that Theophilus believed she was insane. After this meeting, the doctor sided with Theophilus and sentenced Elizabeth to an asylum.

Elizabeth remained locked up for three years until her son was old enough to obtain her release and bring her home. However, after Elizabeth returned home, Theophilus locked Elizabeth in the house and nailed the windows shut. She went from one prison back to another.

Regardless of the medical advice being given or mandates from the church, one overarching belief permeated throughout the centuries—women are property. They may fill a prescribed role in society, fulfill the purpose of procreating the next generation, but they are not entitled to their own personhood. As women began to push back against their social situations and status, they were given the labels and diagnoses of insane and then institutionalized.

Statistics from the National Institute of Mental Health revealed that from 1950-1968, approximately 220,000 more women were hospitalized in state mental asylums than men. Were women really more mentally unstable than men during this time or was their behavior more likely to be labeled a mental illness? It wasn't until 1952 that the American Psychiatric Association no longer considered hysteria a mental health condition. Yet, in 1968, it reappeared in the *Diagnostic and Statistical Manual of Mental Disorders (DSM)-II* before it was removed again in 1980, for good, in the *DSM-III*.

Regardless of class, women were curious about their bodies and sex. Unfortunately, they had no access to medically accurate information and were certainly not allowed to discuss this topic. This reality is depicted when Daphne Bridgerton, from the popular Netflix series, *Bridgerton*, has an awkward pre-wedding night chat with her mother, Violet. Mama Bridgerton sits Daphne down during the wedding reception and uncomfortably stumbles through a weird sex talk.

Daphne's innocent question is reflective of the situation most brides found themselves in on their wedding night during the late Victorian period: "If [this act] is this difficult to discuss, how difficult must it be to perform?" Daphne is eager to understand and tells her mother that she has many more questions. Unfortunately, though much to her mother's relief, those questions are never addressed because it is time for Daphne and her new husband to leave for their honeymoon.

Publicly, this approach of silence and shame to discussing or even understanding sex prevailed for much of the 20th century. However, as women began to enter the workforce and were no longer mere extensions of their husbands, their attitudes towards sex privately began to change. One of the earliest sex researchers, Clelia Mosher, who died in 1940, found that sex was often seen among educated women as a normal desire. Some, of course, worried that they shouldn't enjoy sex too much. Many saw it as a form of intimacy with their spouses, as something natural, and as void of hysterical stereotypes.

With women working and gaining freedom of their own, there was still an intense fear of being sexually active. Sex could result in pregnancy. Birth control didn't become publicly available until the 1960s, so abstinence continued to be a means of birth control. The popular excuse, "Not tonight, honey, I have a headache," was the middle-class mantra among women who didn't want more children.

One must understand that it's not that these women didn't want sex. They didn't want sex that resulted in an unplanned or undesired pregnancy. As a woman who has always had fairly easy access to birth control, I find this an important point to make. So often, women of this era are portrayed as frigid, asexual, and prude.

As someone who has never had to struggle with controlling my fertility, I never even considered the weight these women carried. If they were to give into their sexual desires, whether in the confines of marriage or not, they risked everything. And of all the insights this research has shown me, this was the greatest. This is also something we'll discuss later. But I had to note the significant role that fear played in our foremothers' lives when it came to sex and their bodies.

Despite the "free love" movement of the 1970s, most Americans continued to follow Victorian era norms when it came to sex, making the political and cultural shift back to "traditional family values" in the 1980s much smoother. Pregnancies outside of wedlock were stigmatized at worst, but were considered scandalous in the middle and upper classes. How a woman's body worked, menstruation, and sex were still not publicly discussed.

As a child born during this time, I remember asking questions about these subjects and learning quickly that it was inappropriate to have such curiosities. One time I asked a babysitter what the word "masturbation" meant. She told me she didn't know, so I looked it up in a dictionary. I found it, read the definition, but told her I couldn't find it in there. I knew that, even as a child, talking about this with others made me feel uncomfortable, which meant that there must be something wrong with it.

In an attempt to regain the loosening grip the Church had on sexual behavior, the Evangelical Movement promoted the concept of courting in the late 1990s. Courting involves a young man requesting permission from the father of the girl he wished to court. Courting prohibits the interested couple from being alone and limits physical affection to hugging and holding hands. Dating was seen by many in the Church as contributing to sexual delinquency and promiscuity. The belief that you do not date for fun, you date to find your spouse, permeated youth group culture. And while marriage and family were idealized in these circles, sex was never discussed (other than if you do it and you're not married, you're majorly sinning and probably going to Hell).

I cannot tell you how many women I've worked with who got married and started a family because they felt like it was the "right thing to do." They accepted the belief that sex outside of marriage was wrong and because of this, many ended up settling for a partner out of the fear of not finding one later. They looked around and saw their friends getting engaged and starting families. So they jumped on the bandwagon, hitching theirs to their seemingly best option. Meanwhile, under the surface, freedom and family values were feeling at odds. Stability, it would seem, ultimately won out, but at a great cost.

Everything is Fine

How often have you swallowed your desires or buried your dreams because you felt like it was the right thing to do? You put others' needs before your own. Time and time again. As a mom, I used to be so focused on making my kids happy. Tending to all their needs, completely ignoring mine. "Everything's fine; being a mom is great," I would say with a plastered smile. But deep down, I was so tired. And resentful. And just an unhappy person. Why? Because I wasn't making my joy a priority.

You know what makes for great family values? A happy mom. A fulfilled wife. A woman who has permission, not from others, but from herself, to go after the things that light her up.

It's normal if you don't even know what that is! It's not like we have a history of people asking us what we want.

Now is your chance, your time, to ask yourself these questions. To acknowledge why you may feel a little dead inside. To see that you've been disconnected from yourself.

Toolbox:

- What did I expect to read about at the beginning of this chapter?
- Was I surprised by any of the information?
- What stories resonated the most with me?
- How do I see these women and their roles differently? How do I see myself differently?

3

PURITY & POP CULTURE

"Whenam I going to get a ring?" I asked my mom. (No, I wasn't referring to a wedding ring; I was referring to a different kind of ring, a purity ring.)

"Do you want one?" she replied.

"Yeah, I mean Laney already has one and so does..." I rattled off the names of half the girls in my freshman class.

"Ok, well let's go look for one next time we're at the jewelers," she suggested.

"Dad's not going to do like a special dinner or anything?" I wondered.

"Why would he do a special dinner?" my mom inquired.

Clearly she knew nothing of these special ceremonies. "Mom, don't you listen to anything I say?" I said frustratedly. I swear, she never listens, I thought.

"I don't remember you mentioning a dinner..." she trailed off and went back to doing the dishes.

"Ugh, never mind," I responded in irritation, hopping off the counter I was sitting on. I headed to my room and plopped down on my bed. I guess I'm on my own for this, I thought to myself. Didn't she understand how important my purity was? I was ready to vow my chastity until I found the man God had for me, and she was clueless about the entire thing.

At that moment, my self-righteousness was born.

IF YOU HAVE ABSOLUTELY no idea what I'm talking about, then you probably didn't grow up in purity culture. This was a movement within the Evangelical Christian Church in the mid to late 1990s (though I'm sure it's still prevalent today) where pubescent girls would pledge their sexual purity to their fathers (and families) until their wedding day. This was often signified by the promise ring the girl received from her father. Sometimes the father would take the daughter out on a special dinner date and present her with the ring. She would also sign a pledge that might or might not be signed by a (male) youth pastor from her church as well. Some churches would even (again, some still do) throw purity balls. The ball would be attended by fathers and daughters and would involve the girls publicly pledging (also signing a contract) that they would abstain from sex until marriage.

I never attended a purity ball and my parents never got me a purity ring, but I was steeped deeply in this culture. The expectation was that I wouldn't have sex until I was married. Because girls who did lacked character and a commitment to God and to their family. And the people-pleaser part of me would never allow that to happen.

Despite desperately wanting to remain a virgin until my wedding day, I found myself drawn to the temptations of popular culture. I listened to explicit music that talked about "bangin' on the bathroom floor" and someone's "milkshake bringing all the boys to the yard." I would longingly listen to the songs of Jon B and Boyz II Men about love, passion, and desire. I craved the connections found in those lyrics. But those longings also filled me with shame (I shouldn't be having those desires, right?) so I repressed them.

I often felt torn between two value systems—the one of my faith and the one of the world. I was taught to not conform to the world but to reject it because it would only corrupt me and lead me to a life of sin. Yet, I craved so much of what was in the world (which of course was the problem—desires couldn't be trusted). I would escape into the worlds portrayed in movies and television shows (long before the age of Netflix and streaming) and wonder what life in a public school would be like. I would watch movies like *She's All That, Fear, Cruel Intentions, Clueless,* and the *American Pie* series. I would judge the characters for their lack of morality while simultaneously wishing for an opportunity to be desired and sexualized just like the main characters.

What I didn't realize then was that I longed to be seen. I wanted so badly to be valued. For my intelligence, compassion, humor, and charm. But girls didn't get noticed for those things. I mean sure, you make the honor roll, and your name gets printed on a program. But no one's making movies about that.

Instead, movies are made about smart, "good" girls getting made over and finally noticed by the hot, popular guy. The messages were clear—girls get noticed for being skinny, dressing in the right clothes, and having a nice rack. Girls get noticed for their sexual appeal and social status. Girls in those movies leveraged their looks to get what they wanted. They commodified their sexuality and the boys were happy consumers.

Slut Shaming

One way I preserved my self-righteousness (which was also my social currency) was by creating distance between myself and the "sluts" of my peer group. I went to a small, Christian high school where we had to sign a code of conduct that prohibited drug and alcohol use as well as sexual activity. Going to parties and hooking up with guys was not something you proudly did; in fact, you faced expulsion and shaming your family in the process. But I did play in club soccer and basketball and attended church with girls who didn't have such restrictions or face consequences for the latter.

Despite regularly engaging in sexual activities besides vaginal penetration with my boyfriends, I was not considered a slut or easy. I was able to present my sexuality in a way that was perceived as innocent yet knowledgeable, and most importantly, preserved. This was, of course, in contrast with girls who were promiscuous (which I'm sure I defined as having at least one sexual partner), who lacked moral character, and who were thus subjugated to social sanctions (rightfully so, I believed, because they lacked self-control).

Slut shaming wasn't something that regularly happened in my school. But it was evident throughout the mainstream media and experienced by many women. Nina shared her story with me. One she carried for 23 years. She never told anyone about what happened because she was so filled with shame. When Nina was 15 years old, she started dating a cute and popular boy. One of her friends asked her to check on her house while she and her family went out of town one weekend. Knowing they would have an empty house to themselves, Nina shared this with her boyfriend who suggested they meet up there.

Nina revealed that they started to have sex and it was very painful. She told her boyfriend that it hurt and he told her, "Hang in there, I'm almost done." Nina felt like she couldn't take her consent back, so she just laid there with tears streaming down her face. Afterward, she noticed that she had bled all over her friend's bed. Embarrassed, she told her friend. Nina's friend told everyone what happened, "Nina fucked this guy and bled all over my bed." And to top it off, Nina's boyfriend dumped her the next week and started dating one of her best friends.

Nina's core group of girlfriends began to exclude her. She would be walking down the hallway at school, and someone would say "whore" loudly but not directly to her face. In class, others would make nasty comments like, "If you're the kind of person that stains other people's beds..." Nina faced an abundance of passive aggressive behaviors; for example, suddenly there was no room for her at her friend's lunch table. Nina began to skip school to avoid harassment. One day, she came to school drunk. "Maybe if I lighten up my friends will like me again and think I'm funny; they'll remember the fun me," Nina shared. But that didn't happen. Instead, she got suspended.

Tired of fighting the realities she was facing at school, she decided to embrace the slut title. She would date a guy and sleep with him within the first few weeks. "I was so emotionally desperate for love. I was perpetuating the rumors, acting like I didn't care," she told me.

This trauma affected Nina for over two decades. It prevented her from showing up online in her business because she was afraid of being called a slut by her old crowd. She feared her husband finding out. "What if he thinks I'm just a big slut?" she thought. When I asked Nina whether her boyfriend at the time received any harassment or faced any repercussions, she laughed and said, "Nope, just another virgin he got."

Nina's experience highlights so many realities. Even though all her girlfriends were dating and having sex, none of them were stigmatized as sluts. Sometimes, Nina's friends would flippantly call one another a slut, but it was mainly out of jest— until it wasn't, in Nina's case, and so many other women's. So many women have been traumatized by slut shaming. And yet these women aren't having sex by themselves.

There's typically a male partner in the mix who gets off (literally and figuratively) scot-free. Sure, the term "man-whore" gets thrown around, but it feels more like an oxymoron than an insult. It's another nod to the belief that "boys will be boys" and to the good girl–bad girl dichotomy.

When examining the word *slut*, here is what I found. It is predominantly used by girls who seek male attention and status by slandering other girls. It's the modern-day equivalent of accusing a fellow woman of being a witch three hundred years ago. In fact, the vast majority of individuals who accused women of being witches were girls and young women. We threw our own under the bus and watched silently as they burned at the stake. Slut shaming allows the accuser to move the spotlight onto someone else and reinforce their own self-righteousness.

Because if we can hold on to the belief that we are doing the "right" thing (playing by the rules, adhering to societal messaging, coloring inside the lines), then we'll finally reap the rewards, right? I know that's what I was promised.

But humans are more complicated than that. Doing A does not guarantee you'll get B; yet, that was the messaging so many in my generation received. And when someone chooses to create their own path, to follow their own desires and heart, that feels unsafe to us. So we try and cage them with our words. We isolate them with our actions. We distance ourselves from the "slut" because we're afraid that her choice to forge her own path will be contagious. And we don't want to be like her. Do we?

Lies We've Been Told About Sex

"How do I overcome the shame I have in my marriage?" Ayesha asked, staring at the floor.

"What do you mean?" I asked.

She spoke softly, "Well, I wasn't a virgin when I married my husband, and he was. We both grew up in the church, but I had sex with other boyfriends before him."

"Ok. Is that a problem for you?" I wondered.

She finally made eye contact with me. "What do you mean?" she asked.

"I mean is there a reason you are upset about it? You seem like you're carrying a really big burden," I told her.

She shifted in her seat and then said, "I just always thought it was bad that I'd had sexual partners before my marriage. Is that why I have a higher sex drive than my husband? Is God punishing me because of my choices as a young adult?"

Oh, sweet sister, I thought. I shook my head, "No, no, no," I began. I didn't even know where to begin to address her concerns. I put my hands to my mouth in a prayer pose, briefly closed my eyes, and breathed in deeply. Then I put my hands down and said, "Those are lies. None of them are true. Not one single truth. But before we can accept the truth, the incredible loving truth that can set us free, we have to address those lies. And that's exactly what we're going to do."

HONESTLY, I could write an entire book about the lies we've been sold about sex. They range from the ridiculous to the hysterical to the harmful. Instead, I've compiled the top three. Ones I've faced personally and ones I've spoken to thousands of women about.

It was hard to narrow down these top three. When I asked women about the lies they've been told about sex, many of them stated that it was harder for them to identify the truths they were told.

Let me repeat that. It was harder for most women to think of a truth they were told about sex than a lie. Good night nurse. And we wonder why we have difficulties with this area.

Lie #1: It's my duty as a wife to please my husband. (There's a part B to this too.) My husband deserves access to my body whenever he wants it.

My friend, Sasha, shared with me the only marriage advice she received as a newlywed. "I never talked to my friends about sex. Our church never talked to me about sex in marriage. One day, I was at a friend's house, chatting with a group of women. A woman I very much respected was there and told me that I should 'never say no to my husband.' She was a doctor and a lifelong fellow Catholic, so of course I valued her opinion. I'll never forget her telling me that." Hearing my friend share this with me left me dumbfounded. Is that really the best advice we have for newlyweds?

While I never explicitly received this advice, the message was inferred. It was assumed that men who cheated on their spouses did so because they weren't getting their sexual needs met at home. If you want to keep a man, you keep him happy. And we all know the best way to do that is in the bedroom.

When we deny our spouse access to their pleasure (because we're the vessel that provides that), it creates dissent in the marriage. And that's how the devil gains a foothold. How do you prevent this? By giving your man whatever he wants whenever he wants it. By denying your own needs and concerns. By disconnecting from the discomfort.

The Hard Truth: no one, and I mean absolutely no one on this planet, has a right to your body. You are not property. You are not a possession. That marriage license is not a deed of sale. How other people behave is a reflection of themselves, not you. Now, do I believe that each partner in a relationship is worthy of giving and receiving pleasure? Of course! But that is not born of obligation. It comes from a place of love and longing. If you struggle with meeting your partner's sexual needs, if you struggle with setting and enforcing boundaries, if you struggle with communicating about sex, that is another conversation. However, I would encourage you to determine whether those issues are rooted in this lie.

Lie #2: Masturbation is wrong and shameful.

I remember watching the movie, *Fried Green Tomatoes*, as a girl. I was absolutely mortified at the scene where the main character, Evelyn, shows up to a women's empowerment meeting and the first thing the organizer says is that they're all going to take out a mirror and look at their vaginas. Who does that? WHY would a woman do that, I wondered. And based on Evelyn's reaction of running from the meeting in terror, this belief was reinforced. That's so gross. And yet, that area feels so good. I didn't understand the dichotomy. Why was there such a discrepancy between what we were told and how our bodies were created?

I don't dislike the word *masturbation*, but I find that a lot of women are more open to the term, "self-stimulation." Why? Because masturbation, the word, can conjure up images and feelings of sin and shame.

I want to make an important distinction here. Self-stimulation is the act of stimulating one's own genitals for sexual pleasure. This does not have to occur while using pornography. Do people use pornography while sexually stimulating themselves? Of course. I just want you to be aware of the difference and remind you that you can absolutely engage in self-stimulation without utilizing pornography.

Many receive the message that masturbation is wrong from their church. I fully acknowledge that I am not a pastor or a theologian. I'm just the product of a kindergarten-through-college Christian education and a lifelong Christian. I'm just here sharing my truth, both professionally and personally. Many religious traditions will condemn self-pleasure, or really any pleasure in general. If you find yourself in such a religious tradition, research why those messages are there and what they are based on. And then decide for yourself how you feel about it.

The Hard Truth: the best way to understand your body, including how it responds to certain forms and types of touch, is by exploring it yourself. So many women don't enjoy sex with their partners because they don't enjoy sex with themselves. You don't have to have sex with yourself to enjoy sex with someone else, but I do see a correlation (not causation) here.

If you find yourself hesitant to explore your body sexually, ask yourself why. Where does that belief come from? Is it true? Can I explore my body without lusting or fantasizing about someone else (if that's something I find opposes my religious beliefs)? Am I afraid my partner thinks self-stimulation is wrong? Do I feel comfortable bringing up this topic to discuss with them? Answering these questions is critical to uncovering how you feel about this topic.

Lie #3: Previous sexual experiences outside of marriage are wrong and will impede your married sex life.

In my Christian high school, girls received the message that sex outside of marriage made one "used goods." I remember one girl asking the Family Life Educator during our "sex education" talk, "Shouldn't you test drive a car before you buy it?" The woman looked at the girl, cocked her head and said, "Why would you do that? Wouldn't you trust that God will provide a car that works perfectly well and was built just for you?" Sure, we all thought. I mean that made sense to a bunch of sexually inexperienced teenagers who were told to blindly trust God for everything else. Why not sex too?

Not wanting your future husband to think that you're a

wadded-up piece of paper or a chewed-up piece of gum (both actual illustrations I've heard from numerous Christian women) is a great way to instill the fear of sexual activity into the minds and hearts of young girls. And throwing in the impact it will have (not *could have* because there is no uncertainty in the messaging) on your future union solidifies the decision to keep those legs sealed tight.

Honestly, in all my work and in all the conversations I've had with couples, I've never had someone say, "I'm really affected by the number of people they've slept with." You know what couples care about? Infidelity, hiring prostitutes, high risk sex (e.g., unprotected or stranger sex), no sex. How many people Johnny banged when he was in college does not make it to the top 10 things I've talked to my clients about.

It's helpful to remember that sex is a skill. No one talks about that, but it's really important to realize. Just because you have genitals doesn't mean you know how to use them in a way that gives you the results you're desiring. Unlike most other skills, say baking or communicating or playing basketball, you're not encouraged to put in a lot of practice and learn how to get better at it.

It's also not something that is modeled for you, like those other skills are. Pornography is NOT where you learn how to have sex. Watching porn is like watching NASCAR thinking that's how you'll learn to drive a car.

I do want to make a note about this lie. Former partners can impact your future sex life if there is a trauma or a violated boundary. Those kinds of things are not something you can just shake off. Those experiences can be difficult to move on from and heal without professional help or intention.

The Hard Truth: This messaging is a fear-mongering technique. It's just another way to control women's sexual behavior. No woman wants to endanger her future family, so if we set her up to be a martyr at a young age, then it's a lot easier for her to keep that identity when she's a mother. Control. Control. Control.

Ask Why

"Alright, any questions?" I enthusiastically asked after finishing my talk on How to Talk to Your Kids About Sexuality at the local Mothers of Preschoolers (MOPS) Group. Several women raised their hands.

"Yes," I said and smiled, pointing to a brunette woman at one of the tables.

"Thank you so much for your talk," she said with a smile. "You gave us all a lot to think about. I am wondering, though, how can I keep my kids pure?"

I took a deep breath before I answered her question. I knew her intentions were good, but honestly, I despise that word: *pure*. I was trying to process my feelings toward the question while also respecting her sincere inquiry. "Well," I began, "I'll be honest. I'm not a big fan of the word, *pure*. I find that it sends the message that any sexual activity, however your family defines that, will leave a child feeling impure. Defective. Like they did something wrong. Like they *are* something wrong. And I don't think any of us want our kids feeling that way."

I tried to decide where I wanted to take this answer. Do I address the lasting impacts of sexual shame? Should I bring up the fact that 90% of Americans have sex before they get married? I decided to take a different approach.

"Let me ask you this. What do you want your kids to know about sex? Because as much as we want to control our children's behavior, the truth is we can't forever. At some point, we have to trust our parenting and believe that we've succeeded in raising sexually healthy adults. That we've equipped our kiddos the best we can. But to do that, we have to understand why WE want them to be pure or to delay sex until a certain time period or event. If you're wanting your kids to abstain from sexual activity out of fear, they'll pick up on that and they will carry that burden into their marriage. If you're wanting your children to abstain from sex out of love, find that reason. Find why it matters to you and then find a way to convey that so they'll listen."

A woman from another table spoke up, "I know what that's like," she said looking at the woman and then at me. "My parents never told me about sex or anything about my body or pleasure or consent. I adhered to the church's message that sex before marriage was wrong. It was dirty. I mean, it can't be good if no one talks about it, right?" Other women around the room nodded their heads in agreement.

"Yes!" I replied. "We've been taught to accept these messages from authority as the gospel truth without questioning WHY. Why is sex before marriage wrong? Why are we wanting our kids to be *pure* until they say, 'I do?'"

"Because that's what the Bible says," the woman who asked the original question confidently stated.

I didn't want to get into a theological debate, so I gave my standard response to questions like these. "I'm not a pastor. I'm not a Biblical scholar, so I'm not here to debate the Bible. But here's what I will tell you. The reasons you give to your kids for why you discipline them, why you enforce the rules you do and convey the values you do, they matter. They add up and impact how they see themselves and the world. It's a lot to consider without easy answers, so I encourage you to look at the messages you're receiving, the words you're reading, and decide what they mean for you and your family. I'm in those trenches with you, mamas. I know we're all doing the best we can. And when we know better, we do better. Even when it's hard. Even when it feels scary. Because that's what we do for our kids. And for ourselves."

Toolbox:

- How has purity culture affected how I approach and experience sex?
- How have I participated in slut shaming? How has slut shaming affected me?
- What lies resonate the most? What's preventing me from accepting the truth?
- What do I want my child(ren) to know about sex? How can I empower them with the truth?

4

MIRROR, MIRROR

"Ugh, I look so fat in these jeans," my size-two friend lamented to me.

"I don't think that's possible," I told her.

She waved off my disagreement and continued to look at herself from various angles in the full-length mirror.

HAVE you ever had a conversation like this? I've had multiple, both as the friend complaining about her body and the one trying to convince her friend that she's not fat. No matter how much we try to convince ourselves (or others try to convince us), it seems that our minds are made up. We just don't look the way we think we're supposed to. I find that for many women (me included), this dissatisfaction with our appearances goes deeper, making it hard to really see ourselves. Because, here's the kicker, the mirror we're looking at is distorted.

I remember going to fairs as a kid. They would have this attraction called the House of Mirrors. It was filled with all kinds of weirdly shaped mirrors that reflected silly images of the person standing in front of it. One mirror would make you look two feet tall and four feet wide. Another mirror would make it seem like you had three heads. I would laugh with my friends at all the funny ways we looked in those mirrors.

Unfortunately, most women measure themselves using these kinds of mirrors. We decide who we are and how we feel about ourselves by looking into a mirror that was never meant to determine our outlook, let alone define our worth. And the crazy thing is we don't even realize the mirror we're looking at isn't revealing the whole truth.

So we assume something must be wrong with what we see. The person creating the image must change. Conform. Shrink (physically, spiritually, emotionally, or sexually). We think that by doing this, we will gain the acceptance and approval of others. We hope that others won't walk by and see how hideous we look in the mirror. We fear their judgments because we just want to belong. But in the process of trying to belong, we lose ourselves. We betray our wants and bury our desires. And we keep coming back to the mirror to remind us how wrong we are.

Mirror Work

My client sat at her wooden kitchen table 3,000 miles away from me. The beauty of Zoom allows me to work with individuals anywhere in the world. I shared with Alena that we'd be doing some mirror work today. "Oh good, we can use that mirror over there," I said, pointing to the one behind her.

She turned around to look at the small mirror hanging on her dining room wall.

"You can either take it off the wall and bring it over here for the exercise or just go and stand in front of it," I instructed her. "Whatever you prefer."

"Ok," she said and got up to grab the mirror off her wall. She returned with the mirror in her hand and sat back down.

"Great," I told her. "Now, I want you to take the mirror in a minute and repeat something while looking at yourself. It's important that you maintain eye contact with yourself. Ok?" I confirmed.

"Got it," she confidently said.

"Alright. I want you to tell yourself, 'I love you. I am worthy of love. I deserve good things,'" I said and nodded my head as an indication for her to begin.

"Ok," she calmly replied. She picked up the mirror and began, "I..." she paused and cleared her throat. "I...love...you," she slowly spoke the words, "I can't. I can't say this," she said with tears streaming down her face. "Why can't I say them?" she longingly asked me.

My face fell to sadness because I knew why she couldn't speak those words. "Because you don't believe them," I told her. "Your body is tired of pretending."

"But if someone asked me if I loved myself, I would tell them that of course I did. I know I deserve good things. So why can't I say that now without breaking down in tears?"

"Because," I began, "because you realized that you've been living as a fraud. We don't believe words just because we say them. We can't just think our way into loving ourselves. We have to feel it to believe it. We have to live it to learn it. One of my favorite quotes is by Father Richard Rohr. He says, 'We do not think ourselves into new ways of living, we live ourselves into new ways of thinking.'"

I went on to share, "My dad used to read a lot of books. He would consume them within a couple days and then move onto the next one. Sometimes he would share with me what he was reading—a recent diet trend, a leadership approach, how to be a better parent. The thing was that he never really applied what he learned. He thought he could think his way into his life being different. What he didn't realize was that he had to make the changes for his brain to start seeing things differently. He had to experience the change so that his body could begin integrating the learnings too. This is what Father Richard Rohr meant with his profound words. Thinking doesn't make us experience things differently. Only living differently can do that. Thankfully, you're at the best place. Because your mind and body are on the same side. They're ready to begin to dig deep and look at the other lies you've been telling yourself. No more pretending, ok?"

My client nodded her head in agreement and wiped the tears from her face, "No more pretending."

Would You Choose Beautiful?

One afternoon, when my kids were little and I was deep in the stage of diapers and potty training and toddler meltdowns, my daughter's words stopped me in my tracks. Man, were those tough years. Honestly, it all feels like a blur when I look back. My husband was doing his medical fellowship, and I had three kids under five. I spent most days exhausted, questioning my value as a mother and a woman. But I will never forget where I was when my daughter told me in her sweetest little 3-year-old voice, "Mommy, I'm beautiful."

I stopped loading the car and turned to her, a little surprised, honestly, with her statement. I stared at her in her pink tutu and mismatched shoes. I marveled at her confidence and smiled as she squeezed her favorite stuffed penguin. I wish I could tell you that my heart was exploding with pride. That I thought, wow, that's incredible that she sees herself with such love. No, that's not what entered my mind. Instead, I thought, what if someone hears her say that? What if someone thinks she's being arrogant or doesn't agree with her?

You see, that is the kind of conditioning that runs deep in us. The kind of messaging that keeps a highly educated progressive mother from fully accepting a profound statement of love from her toddler daughter. This conditioning is so great that when my gift from above spoke such truth, her truth, I worried about what others would say and do. I truly believe that our children are our greatest teachers. It's God's way of reminding us that we don't have it all figured out; and honestly, we never will. And that moment was a perfect reminder for me.

Because I have been intentional with my parenting, I knew that how I responded to my daughter's statement mattered. My conditioning wasn't her burden to bear. This cycle didn't have to continue with her. So I pushed aside those thoughts that questioned my little girl's truth. Instead, I told her, "I hope you always believe that, and you tell yourself that every day. Because you are beautiful. Inside and out." She smiled and skipped to her side of the car, still squeezing her penguin, "I know."

If you were about to walk into Target, and you noticed two doors with the labels "Beautiful" and "Average" above them, which one would you walk through? What if no one was around? What about someone you love so deeply like your child or your mother? What door would you want them to walk through? This premise was presented by the company Dove in their Choose Beautiful commercial. It's a powerful commercial to watch, but even more powerful to consider what you would choose.

I would love to say that this same daughter would walk through the door labeled Beautiful. But the truth is, I don't know. She's deep into her tweens and I wonder at what point our girls (though I'm aware this happens with boys as well) lose that innate love of themselves. I've seen statistics stating that approximately 50% of 13-year-old girls are unhappy with their body. And that number grows to roughly 75% by the time girls hit 17. I won't even go into the statistics on disordered eating among adolescents.

Mirror, Mirror

In college, I would often visit a group of my friends who lived off campus in a split-level house. At the top of the first level, a full-length mirror stood, propped against the stair railing at a weird angle. One day I asked about this mirror, "Don't you think it's an odd place for a mirror? Why is it slanted like that?"

One of my friends remarked confidently, "Oh, that's our skinny mirror!"

"Skinny mirror?" I asked.

"Yeah," my other friend said. "The way it's tilted makes you look skinny. So when we walk by it, it makes us feel better about how we look."

I didn't know how to respond. Was it really that simple, I wondered. Could it be that simple?

In a world full of camera filters and facial fillers, it can feel like who you are, just as you are, is never enough. Because it's not enough when we are comparing ourselves to a distortion. Images that have been cropped and photoshopped.

It's daunting to fathom how much our society values beauty. Tall, but not too tall; thin, but not anorexic thin; large breasts; clear, blemish-free skin; voluminous hair—I could go on, but you get the idea.

Having these things or even desiring to have these things

isn't bad. But it's important to understand why they're valued. You see, no one explained to me growing up that most of these characteristics conveyed fertility, and having a fertile partner guaranteed you'd pass your genetic material on to the next generation. Large breasts meant you could feed your baby. A good height and weight meant you were more apt to survive a sprint away from predators. Clear skin indicated a sign of good internal health. A curvy waist meant you had good hips to carry and push a baby out. When you break it down, it makes sense why these things are valued in society. It's a throwback to our ancestors. It's even why popular cartoon characters have such big eyes (they externally represent the ovaries, which means lots of eggs to fertilize).

Bottom line: our society values the propagation of its species, and it really doesn't care how it communicates that to us. Companies don't care whether their messages cause us to judge ourselves out of fear. Fear that we're not thin enough, strong enough, pretty enough, or supple enough. And fear is highly contagious, which is what companies are banking on. Because the more afraid we are, the more likely we are to consume a product that eases that fear.

Governments need their people to make tiny future citizens who pay taxes and consume products. And with a digital commerce and entertainment literally in the palm of our hands, companies are able to communicate these messages a billion times over. Unfortunately, they really don't care whether it hurts our self-esteem in the process (because they probably have a product for that anyway).

Thankfully, companies have been more inclusive in their messaging, representing diverse body types, skin colors, and gender expressions. But marketing has a long way to go. In the meantime, knowing this is what companies are targeting in their messaging is, I find, really helpful. They are speaking to us at our most primitive level, which of course, also applies to messaging on sexual behavior.

"So good news," I told my client. "We're basically set up to fail from the beginning, so just keep that in mind the next time you get down on yourself about not being interested in sex."

"What do you mean," Rian asked.

"Think about the messaging you've received about the type of woman you need to be," I said.

"Oh, yeah," she stated, "I need to be thin but have big boobs and a nice ass. I need to be sexually innocent but also be a vixen."

"Yep," I agreed. "Essentially, find the balance between what Ludacris said, 'a lady in the street but a freak in the bed.'"

She laughed and said, "Oh piece of cake."

WHAT LUDACRIS, the famous rapper, represents with his lyrics is what scholars refer to as the Madonna–whore dichotomy. This polarization presents women as chaste, pure Madonnas (not the 1980s singer; I'm talking about the virgin here) as "good" against seductive, promiscuous (who gets to define what that is?) as "bad." This is just another example of the patriarchy's attempt to regulate women's sexual behavior. And of course, this is reflected to us in popular culture from the way shampoo is marketed (looking at you, Herbal Essences) to who can work at a certain store in a shopping mall (ahem, Abercrombie & Fitch).

Why does any of this matter? Because it affects how we show up. How we value ourselves. I want to pull back the curtain so you can see that it's not the great and powerful Oz calling the shots. It's centuries of programming and prejudices that have kept us—kept our sexuality, our passion, and creativity—regulated and repressed. And not knowing that truth prevents us from truly being set free.

It's not just *our* own chains. It's the chains that bound our mother, and her mother, and her mother before that, times a thousand. When we realize the collective pain and trauma that have been hidden from us, we realize why our burden is so friggin' heavy. Then maybe, we can finally stop blaming ourselves for being so weak. If we only knew it wasn't just our suffering we've been carrying this whole time.

One of the ways I was intentional about combatting poor body images with my children was by outlawing the "f" word in our house. No, I don't mean that "f" word—*fat*. No one, even visitors, were allowed to use that word in our house. I refused to degrade myself, my body, in front of my children. Even though I struggled with my own body image, I never talked about it in front of my children. I never pinched the fat on my side in front of them. I never complained about my wrinkles. I never talked about going on a diet or needing to lose weight. Those were my burdens to carry, not my children's.

I did take them with me to the gym. I did talk about needing to reduce the amount of sugar I ate. I did talk about creating a balanced plate that could fuel my body. I did share with them my running goals. But never from a place of fear. I was determined to model a healthy and active lifestyle. That doesn't mean I didn't struggle with the number on the scale because in complete honesty I did, and to some extent still do. I've mostly made peace with my body, but sometimes those parts of me that think I should be thinner and younger looking are loud. And that's ok because I know how to work through it.

When we micromanage our bodies, when we are raised to worry and starve, we shut off the world of sensuality, which is of course tied to pleasure. And inspiration. And sexuality. We divorce ourselves from our bodies because the idea of being fully present in them is just too much.

You may be thinking, but what if I don't micromanage my body? What would happen then?! That's a great question. One I remember asking my nutritionist years ago. She told me that I could love my body AND still work towards my goals of being healthier. That truth totally changed my life. Because I thought I had to hate my body into change. I thought I had to shame myself for even wanting a piece of cake. I thought I had to be disgusted at myself when I looked in the mirror.

But what I have found, both personally and professionally, is that nothing good and nothing lasting comes from a place of hate.

A Powerful Woman

"What do you do for fun?" I asked Jenny.

She looked at me in confusion and then laughed. "Fun? I don't have time for fun," she said seriously.

I nodded my head because I remember speaking those words so many years ago. "Ok," I started. "What about hobbies?"

She laughed again, "Are you serious? I don't have any hobbies."

I leaned forward in my chair a little. "Alright. What are you passionate about?"

She pursed her lips together and considered the question. About 20 seconds went by, "Um, I...hmm. I don't know."

I nodded my head again, "Ok. What brings you joy? What are things that you enjoy doing?"

She began to shake her head and said despondently, "I don't...I don't know. How do I not know? How sad is it that I have no idea what I'm passionate about or that I have no time for fun? What is this life I'm living?"

"Well," I responded, "it's actually a lot more common than you think. We're not really raised to be in connection with our passion. That's beaten out of us at a pretty young age. 'Find a job that makes you a lot of money. Marry the right person. Have kids. Be a slave to the grind.' And we accept it. Hook. Line. And sinker. And then we're caught in the endless cycle of obtaining and maintaining a 'successful' life."

"Yes," she agreed. "But how do I find out what I am passionate about? How do I have fun?"

I smiled, "You have to start believing that you're deserving of a life filled with fun and joy. A life full of freedom."

I could see my client moving in her chair, turning her body a little away from me.

"Does that make you uncomfortable?" I asked her.

She could tell that I picked up on her body language. She crossed her legs and said,

"Honestly? Yes. The idea of creating a 'life of freedom' terrifies me."

"Good. It should," I stated.

She looked at me confused.

"Do you know what scares society?" I paused. "A powerful woman," I told her. "And why do you think that is?"

"I don't know," she replied.

"Because a powerful woman is free. She doesn't live a life of obligation. She makes decisions based on her values. She spends her time doing things that are life-giving. A powerful woman isn't someone who is willing to be controlled by societal expectations or social norms. When a woman prioritizes her wants and needs, it creates a ripple effect of peace and love around her. And it shows the next generation that you *can* create a life you truly love."

She looked at me and wondered, "Is that really possible?"

I smiled and said, "You tell me."

. . .

A MORE AUTHENTIC way of living *is* possible. Authentic living isn't living in a fantasy world. It's about identifying your values and aligning your energy, beliefs, and time in accordance with them. Authentic living is incorporating honesty into your interactions with others. It's respecting your boundaries and limits. It's about letting go of the need to prove anything to anyone. It truly is a life of freedom.

Consider what we tell our kids. "You need to work hard in school, play three sports, play a musical instrument, learn at least one foreign language, volunteer regularly, and go to church so that you can

- get into a good college (take on a significant burden of debt)
- get a high paying job (so you can work all the time)
- marry someone who makes good money too (so you never see each other)
- buy a great house in a great neighborhood (hello, more debt)
- drive a safe but appealing car (more debt)
- have children (so you have no energy or time to enjoy seeing them and then you feel guilty about it)

And this may lead to anxiety, depression, neglected physical health, autoimmune disorders, financial stress, and an overall dissatisfaction with life. Our bodies push back when we are living out of alignment with who we truly are."

We conform because we don't know any other way. Despite being highly educated, I never considered another way was possible. But there is! However, that new life, the one filled with joy and passion, will cost you your old one. And that can feel scary because it is. But it's also incredibly freeing. And fun. And full of adventure.

And that is the message I'm giving to my kids.

Your Turn

Before you go to the next chapter, I want you to do one thing for me. I want you to find a mirror. And I want you to stare at that beautiful face of yours. The one with a few chin hairs, wrinkles, blemishes—yep that's the one. And I want you to take your hands and softly cup the sides of your face.

Now imagine that face 30, 40, 50-plus years ago. See that little girl. Find her in that face of yours. For you are that little girl. That little girl realized. That little girl who dreamed and laughed and sang and danced like it didn't matter. Nothing mattered to her because she was free. Free to be whatever she wanted to be. Whoever she wanted to be. And along the way, that little girl got lost, got beaten down. Took on burdens that were far too heavy for her little shoulders. And she forgot what it was to dream and dance and laugh and sing.

That little girl is still inside you. That little girl is still you. Find her. Set her free.

Toolbox:

- Do I truly believe that I am deserving of a life filled with fun and joy? A life full of freedom? What's stopping me if I don't?
- Would I choose beautiful? Would the other women in my life? How can I be an example to other women and girls (including the next generation) and empower them to choose beautiful?

- What is one thing I can change (big or small) so I can live a more authentic life?
- Complete the mirror work exercises and consider that little girl. How can I protect her? Love her? Set her free?

PART II

LIGHT THE MATCH

When I was a kid, I loved playing with matches. For the record, I was very responsible with them. Because I knew their power. I had seen the destruction that happens when someone is careless with their flame. My mother had instilled a great fear of lighting candles, and still to this day, it's hard for me to light one without hearing her scolding voice about their dangers.

For those few seconds when I lit a match, I felt powerful. A slight rush would permeate my body. Maybe it was a sense of rebellion. Maybe it was a sense of excitement. Whatever the reason, it was intoxicating.

Pleasure feels much the same. And that's what Part 2 is all about: deciding why you're on this journey, determining that pleasure is your right, understanding how your body experiences pleasure, and of course, embodying that.

5

PERMISSION FOR PLEASURE

"You mentioned on the phone that you're struggling with leaving your marriage. Can you tell me more about that?" I asked Misha.

"Yeah, so..." she began, sighing before her next words. "My husband is just a jerk. He drinks a lot and then he gets mean and cranky. Of course, he doesn't see it as a problem. It's been going on for years now, and I'm just to the point where I can't take it anymore."

"Ok," I nodded my head. "So what's stopping you from leaving?" I asked.

"Well, other than trying to single-parent my four boys and starting over on a teacher's salary, I keep wondering, who's going to want me, you know?" she said.

"That's a fair concern," I told her. "Let me ask you this. Would you want you?"

Misha looked at me and tilted her head to the side, "I..." she began and then stopped. "I don't know, honestly. I mean would you want a divorced mom of four in her early forties?" she asked me.

"Is that only how you see yourself?" I asked her.

"I don't know," she said, shaking her head. "I've never really thought about myself apart from being a mom or a wife or a teacher."

"That's because society likes to define us by what we *do* instead of who we *are*," I told her.

"So how do I become someone that someone else would want?" she asked me.

I smiled and said, "By being that someone to yourself first."

WHEN I'M WORKING with clients, I'm aware of the layers that need to be pulled back. A client will present with one issue—in Misha's case, the struggle to leave her miserable marriage. But there are always several layers underneath this. These layers often prevent us from accessing those core issues or core wounds. For this reason, individuals can get stuck on those outer layers, where the head knowledge is.

For Misha, she was stuck on the outer layers where she was able to identify that she didn't want to be in an unhappy marriage. She understood the logic of it, but she couldn't go deeper into the feelings of it. So she stayed stuck in the knowledge layer, unable to integrate the learnings into her life, unable to take action.

This state of being overwhelmed is normal. It's why reading a book on codependency or personal empowerment isn't usually enough. When knowledge stays in the brain, it doesn't permeate the rest of our body.

Thoughts are the language of the brain, but feelings are the language of the body. This is the reason you can't just talk yourself into calming down or having better sex or a hundred other things. Our bodies don't understand thoughts. They communicate via vibrations (e.g., music), movement, breath, feeling, and attachment. This is why traditional talk therapy isn't that effective. Because it only addresses one component of our total selves.

When we ignore our bodies and major networks like our nervous system, it's like fighting with one arm behind our back. Can we win that way? Sure. But it's a helluva lot harder. And that's usually why most people haven't seen "success" in their lives. If you've ever struggled with losing or gaining weight, accomplishing anything physical (e.g., running a marathon or climbing a mountain), or achieving (e.g., promotions or increased salaries), it's usually because the body isn't on board with your goals.

When we're able to speak to the brain *and* body, things start to change. Our systems start communicating with each other. Everyone gets on board with the new vision. When you've been disconnected from your body, it's like having a cut telephone wire. You can talk and plan all you want, but there's no one on the other end. Those wires have been severed. So it's normal to be frustrated with your lack of progress and to feel lonely in your longings.

Now imagine that you're able to reconnect that phone line. Your brain and body are back online; they're able to communicate with each other. Hooray! But things don't suddenly become glorious. There's still "damage" that needs to be repaired. Damage (low self-esteem, feelings of unworthiness, and of being unlovable) from our lived experiences and limiting beliefs about ourselves and the world.

Instead of tending to the marred wires (the internal work), we focus our energies on buying a new phone (the external issues we face). Or we concentrate on a new house to put our new phone in. We buy the best phone service, so we can prove that we're good at what we do, that we're capable because we have more than enough around us. And all the while, we're neglecting the most important aspect—the wires, which connect us to ourselves.

If it's just a simple wire repair, why don't we just get it done? Because change is scary! Facing ourselves, our past, our hurts, and our shortcomings takes work. It's a whole lot easier to spend time on the things that we think matter to others. To avoid the truth that we feel broken and disconnected. To pretend like everything's ok because if we admit that it's not, then maybe the house of cards we've spent our whole life meticulously building will come crashing down. So we press on, plastering on a smile and a can-do attitude. And we avoid the mirror at all costs because we're afraid that we might catch a glimpse of who we believe we really are.

Stop and Smell the Roses

Growing up, I remember hearing the phrase, "stop and smell the roses." It was often used as an expression for someone who just dilly-dallied and didn't use their time wisely. Someone who chose a slower pace instead of powering through. Who chose rest instead of productivity. I seriously wondered what was wrong with those people? I mean who has the time to stop and smell the roses?

So, I'll ask you—when was the last time you stopped and smelled the roses? Or really any type of flower? I think back to how I would have answered that question in my early twenties. It differs greatly from how I would answer that today.

In all honesty, I probably wouldn't have even noticed the roses. Maybe for their beauty, their aesthetic offering, but never as an opportunity to rest and reflect or appreciate the pleasure they could bring me.

Let's do a quick little exercise. I want you to imagine a beautiful blooming rose right in front of you. Maybe it's bright pink or a deep red or a vibrant yellow. Now, imagine putting that rose to your nose, feeling its silky petals against your nostrils. Take a deep breath (unless of course you're allergic, and then I do not advise this). Now, observe how your body reacted. Did you smile as you inhaled? Did you feel a warmth in your chest or belly? Did a tingle expand through your arms?

When we are intentional, we don't just smell the rose in our nose. We *experience* its scent throughout our entire body. That one small seemingly insignificant moment has the power to permeate our body at the deepest level. And the more often we engage in these minor acts of meaning, the more we reconnect that severed line. We choose presence over numbing. And the more we do that, the easier it is to be in our bodies and fully experience pleasure. Fully experience life.

Do This for You

"So, tell me, what led you to reach out to me?" I asked LaQuesha.

"Um," she began sheepishly. "I've just been having some problems that you may be able to help with."

Sensing her hesitancy, I asked, "Can you tell me a little bit about what's been going on that made you finally decide you wanted help?"

"Sure," she said with a sigh. "I'm just never really interested in having sex and it's causing problems in my marriage."

"What kind of problems," I asked her.

"We just argue a lot. He tells me that he's tired of being 'rejected all the time.' That I never want sex and he needs it. It's just exhausting. So then I just end up having sex with him so we'll stop arguing about it. And that tides him over for a while. Until the cycle starts back over," she shared.

I nodded my head and said, "This is really common among women in committed relationships, especially long-term ones. First, I want you to know that you're not alone. I've talked with thousands of women who feel this exact same way and struggle with the same cycle."

Hearing that made LaQuesha smile slightly.

"Second," I continued, "I want you to know that if you don't want to have sex, then you don't need to have it. Like, if you need a permission slip that says, 'I can say no to sex,' I will happily write you one."

LaQuesha laughed.

"I know that sounds silly, but I'm being one hundred percent serious," I said. "You do not have to do anything sexual if you don't really want to. Even if that means your husband gets upset. Even if that means he nags you about it. Ok?"

LaQuesha's shoulders dropped and she let out a sigh. She asks, "But isn't it easier if I just give him what he wants?"

"Easier for who?" I asked her.

"For me," she stated.

"Let me get this straight," I told her, looking at her beautiful brown eyes starting to fill with tears. "Rather than tell him no, is it easier for you to submit your body to someone who is supposed to love and cherish you even though you have no desire to have your body used for his pleasure?"

Tears began to pour down LaQuesha's face.

"Every time you do that," I continued. "Every time you push away the ability to advocate for yourself by acquiescing to his demands, a part of your spirit, your light, shrinks. Every time you give in to the short-term because it feels easier, you make the long-term more difficult for you. You're not just losing the battles. You're losing the war."

"So what am I supposed to do then?" she asked me.

I smiled and said, "Find the spark inside of you. Reclaim your pleasure and desires. Believe that you deserve more."

I CAN'T TELL you how many women have reached out to work with me because of the insistence of their husband. The husband sees his wife with a problem (or even as THE problem) that needs fixing.

And I don't blame him. Based on everything he's been "taught" about sex and women and pleasure, of course he sees his wife as needing a solution. And to be honest, he's partially right. The issue does lie with her, but not quite how he sees it.

The problem is that LaQuesha, and so many others, have become disconnected from pleasure. Maybe, once upon a time, kissing, fondling, and sex were pleasurable.

Now, it's just a chore with the added societal pressure of performing. Stress has hijacked her brain, triggering the sympathetic nervous system which diverts energy and attention (i.e., blood flow and oxygen) away from the reproductive system. This results in a decrease in physical arousal. So now neither LaQuesha's brain nor body are on board. But she gives in anyway. To keep the peace. To meet her husband's needs. For a hundred other reasons. And she hopes that this will be enough. So she can rest or just get back to doing the things she wants to do.

Pleasure Practice

Let me ask you another question—what do you need right now? What one thing could make you feel just 5% better right now (or in the immediate future)? These are questions that form the foundation of what I call a Pleasure Practice.

Incorporating a Pleasure Practice may feel scary. If you're not used to being in your body, suddenly doing so can feel overwhelming. You may be wondering, "but Courtney, I'm always in my body. Like I can't leave it." And yes, you may not be able to physically leave your body until your final breath, but you can disconnect from it in many ways.

Some of the most common ways I see people disconnect are through substances (food, alcohol, or drugs), success (overworking or working out obsessively), sex (you can go through the motions of sex with your body but be elsewhere with your mind), gambling, and shopping.

These behaviors allow us to escape mentally and physically. They provide dopamine hits that create a reward circuit that causes our body to crave more. This then results in a harmful cycle that many don't know how to find a way out of. When we are brave enough to stop these cycles, to cease the numbing and choose to intentionally listen to our bodies, we begin to reconnect that phone line. We cut away the tangled mess that prevented us from being truly in our bodies, that interfered with our ability to feel and experience, and connect with who we are.

Developing a Pleasure Practice does not have to be difficult or elaborate. In fact, it's meant to give you an easy win. For those of you who grew up believing that self-care or putting your needs before others was selfish, this may require some work on your mindset to feel comfortable. The more you complete your Pleasure Practice, the easier it becomes, and I truly believe it will allow you to get the most out of this life.

If you're feeling overwhelmed with creating a Pleasure Practice, here's one of my favorites: taking a nap. Naps allow me to rest and recharge. And when I wake up from my nap, I'm more grounded and present throughout my day. I make this a Pleasure Practice by paying attention to how I am feeling as I wake up, by tuning into my body and mind in that moment.

Pleasure Practices can be anything from playing a board game to gardening to going for a hike or walk to taking a bath or getting a massage or eating a piece of dark chocolate or sitting quietly with a cup of your favorite beverage. The intention is to incorporate fun, joy, presence, or pleasure into your life. I recommend doing this once a week.

If you follow the moon and planet cycles, I would encourage you to identify your Moon Sign (where the moon was when you were born) and tune into that energy to help nourish this part of you. For example, if you are a Pisces Moon, you may find that being by water (going for a swim, going for a walk by the water, taking a bath) fills your cup. If you're unsure what your Moon Sign is, there are numerous free astro calculators online that will help you discover it.

Establishing a Pleasure Practice isn't just another thing to add to your to-do list. I promise it serves a purpose. See, these actions, the ones that bring you joy and happiness, connect you directly to the most powerful part of yourself. But maybe that idea seems so far off right now.

For many years, I just wanted to light my to-do list on fire. I was so tired of the daily grind. The demands and "must dos." Maybe that's you right now. You have a million things to do and you hate (or resent) just about every one of them. Now, imagine for a moment, that you were looking at your to-do list and you *actually* wanted to check off the things to do. Not because you merely wanted them done and off your list. But because you looked forward to experiencing them. I'm serious. I want you to close your eyes, well after you read this sentence, and picture a to-do list filled with things that bring you joy.

Not all of these items need to be titillating and fun. It's about seeing your to-do list as an opportunity to invite intention into your life and infuse it with some pleasure and lightness. What if your to-do list was about experiencing the things that you already *have* to do, and you were able to find ways to bring them to life?

When we tap into our energetic body, we open ourselves to receiving. In theory, receiving seems awesome. "Yes, I want to receive more good things!" But if it doesn't feel safe in our body to receive, if we have a history of opening ourselves up to others and getting hurt, if we have a history of abuse or trauma, then it's a lot harder to be in that receiving mode, no matter what good things are coming our way.

I want you to imagine a beautiful flower in full bloom with its soft petals completely open. To see the beauty of that flower, it must open. But when it opens itself up to bloom, it also loses its protection. The flower is safer when it's all tucked in and closed up.

You are this beautiful flower, my friend. When you close

yourself off, when you put on your protective armor, you better believe you don't feel the pain as much. But that action comes at a cost because then you can't feel the love and joy and excitement that life has for you.

I know that it can feel dangerous to create a life you love—because how can you be sure it will actually last? You could get disappointed. You could get hurt. And I'm not going to lie to you and tell you that you won't. Because you will. You will ache and cry and long for things that are no longer possible. And then you will realize that those feelings are part of the human experience. You'll begin to see that you are strong and brave and loved.

Both can be true at the same time. Sadness and love. Despair and hope. And then you will remember that deep inside you is a great strength. One that allows you to find your way back home. Back to who you are.

Starting Point

Pleasure doesn't need to start in the bedroom. Honestly, it really needs to start outside of it. It must be realized within ourselves because once it is, we can find and feel pleasure just about anywhere in our lives. Unfortunately, when I work with someone who struggles with finding joy and fun and play in life, I see that affecting their sex life as well. And when we're unhappy and just going through the motions, we disembody, just like that tired mama at bedtime.

Sadly, that's where I see a lot of women today. They are disconnected and dissatisfied emotionally and sexually in their marriages. Initially, they married their partner out of some sort of attraction, but ultimately they sought out matrimony for stability. What I'm seeing is that women in their late 30s to mid-40s are having a hard time seeing their stable partners as sexy.

And because they don't see themselves as sexy either, it's a recipe for infrequent sexual encounters.

What's interesting is that unlike previous generations, dissatisfied women are taking action. Many are filing for divorce because they can't imagine a lackluster marriage for another minute. When these women do come to their husbands with their concerns, they're often met with resistance. The men don't want to change (I know this isn't the case for all men). They're happy with the way things are. Sometimes, there will be an effort to change, but because these men lack the motivation, it is often short-lived. Once again, the woman finds herself frustrated and disconnected.

"IF MY HUSBAND could see my face during sex, he'd be appalled," Zoe said.

"What do you mean?" I asked her.

"I just..." she began. "I'm just to the point where I look at the calendar and I'm like, you know, it's been a while, we should probably have sex, so I do. But I don't really want it."

I asked, "Do you feel like your sexual desire has decreased? We've been dealing with a lot in society right now and that can..."

"I don't really want sex with *him*," she interjected.

"Ok," I said. "Tell me about that."

"It's not that I don't love him or find him attractive. It's just he's so...I don't know...boring, I guess? I mean he's a great dad and..." she trailed off.

"But he's not doing it for you anymore?" I asked.

"No!" she exclaimed. "He's not. And so when we're having sex, I'm just going through the motions and I'm kind of disgusted with myself for doing that. And it's hard to hide that feeling so if the lights were on while we did it, he'd see my facial expression."

I nodded, "I get it." I paused and then asked, "Do you feel like you're settling in your sex life?

She sighed, "Yeah, I guess I do."

"What about other areas?" I asked. "Are you settling in other areas of your life?"

She laughed. "I feel like my mantra is 'it's fine; everything's fine.'"

"Do you want things to just be fine?" I asked her.

She shrugged her shoulders. "I don't know. It just feels like it's so much work to get it above that 'fine' line, you know?"

I nodded my head and smiled, "Well, that's 'cause it is. At first I mean. Anytime we try to take a different path than the one we've been taking, there's some resistance and that feels like work. Our brains don't like change; they like predictability." I paused. "Let me ask you this, do you think *you're* worth the effort? Worth the work it takes to stop settling?"

She considered my question and said, "Honestly, I don't know. I want to say, 'yes.' I feel like that's the right answer, but I don't know."

"Would you be willing to find out?" I asked her.

She laughed, "I mean I guess. What have I got to lose?" she jokingly said.

With a straight face I looked her in her eyes and said, "Everything. And that's how you gain what you want."

For homework, I asked Zoe to consider what she wanted out of life. I told her to list it all out. To really dig deep and ponder the pleasures this life has to offer. When she came back the next week, do you know what was on her list? A single word-joy. I've done this exercise numerous times with clients from all walks of life. It is one of the hardest things for women to do. If I were to ask them what they want for their kids or their loved ones, they could fill an entire page on the spot with experiences and achievements. But when it comes to what *they* want, I'm usually presented with a blank page.

But the thing that saddens me the most when they bring back that empty page is the shame that accompanies it. Their shoulders are hunched, their gaze is low, and their head is hung. "I didn't know what to write," they say, defeated. "Of course, you don't," I tell them confidently. This causes them to perk up a little. "No one has ever given you the permission to dream big for YOU. No one has allowed you to serve a purpose unless it's in relation to others—your spouse, your kids, your job," I tell them. And then I take their paper and I write Permission Slip across it and hand it back to them.

This is your permission slip. You have permission to dream big. To do whatever the hell you want. To live a life of freedom. To stop being bogged down by obligation and expectation. To try something new and fail. I mean fail real big. Because failure is not to be feared. Living a life where you are stuck in the same place and never take risks is a hell of a lot scarier than trying something and not getting the results you wanted. Failure is feedback. If you make it mean something more (I'm a bad person; I'm worthless; I can't do anything), that's your inner critic trying to keep you playing small (really, they have the best of intentions in trying to keep you safe). And that's the issue that needs to be addressed, not your unsuccessful actions.

But please, for the love of all things good, don't sell yourself short. Decide that you have the right to discover and choose what it is that you want. To explore your desires and pursue your pleasures. And if you ever wonder whether you're really allowed to do this, remember this permission slip. Remember that you are the only owner of this one life. Make it great, girl.

Toolbox:

- Create a Pleasure Practice. How can I establish my Pleasure Practice and make it a priority?
- How do I disembody? Where am I just going through the motions (on autopilot)?
- Write out a permission slip to yourself. Be specific. What are you giving yourself permission for?

6

COMPLEXES & BODIES

"I don't really like it when my spouse comes up from behind me when I'm in the kitchen and grabs me," Shia told me.

"Why is that?" I asked.

"I don't know," she said, as she scrunched her face. "I just, I don't know. I guess it just bothers me."

"Which is totally fine if it does," I began. "Anytime something bothers me or annoys me or makes me angry, I like to understand why that is. Let me ask you this. Growing up, did your parents show much affection toward each other?"

Shia tilted her head, considering the question. "Well, not really. But now that you mention it, I remember my mom always shooing my dad's hands away anytime he would try and squeeze her butt or linger too long for a kiss."

I nodded my head and smiled. I was hoping she was seeing the connection.

"Oh my gosh," she exclaimed. "Wow. I can't believe I never thought about that." Shia sat back in her seat processing her realization.

"It's not that you are recreating your childhood, but in a way you kind of are," I said. "When healthy, loving affection isn't modeled, our brains take note. When women are seen as the objects of desire, we receive the message that we are at the whim of our partner's passions. And for so many generations it wasn't safe to speak up and say, 'You know, I'm not comfortable with that, or I don't appreciate being touched this way.' But that's a rare conversation we have with our partner, with ourselves or even with our kids."

Shia sighed, "I just never thought of it that way. I never put much weight onto these interactions, and yet I find that these kinds of encounters have really caused me to resent my spouse and withdraw from her sexually."

I replied, "Well, you're not alone in that. Not even a little."

MANY OF THE women I work with have been conditioned to be passive when it comes to pleasure. Orgasm or ecstasy have often been the byproducts of sexual encounters and not the original intent. And I believe a lot of that is due to what's modeled for us in our homes growing up.

I want you to think back to how affection was shown in your household. Even if you didn't grow up in a "traditional family" with a mom and a dad, how did you see the adults in your life display affection? Was your dad the one trying to initiate play with your mom only to be shut down because she had "other things to do?" Was your mom the one who made sure your dad kissed her hello and goodbye?

It may not seem like the behaviors of your parents really matter, but they actually do. Our brain registers these behaviors as normal, acceptable, and predictable. And even if, logically, we don't want to recreate them in our adult life, it ends up happening because that's the software that's been input. Want to change the output? Change the software.

How do you change the software? First, by taking inventory of the program you're running. Examining where your beliefs and worldviews originated. And then deciding whether you want to trade them in for different ones. Let's take pleasure for example. Were you given permission to pursue pleasure? To go after the things that brought you joy? That fostered your creativity? That inspired you? Or were you told that you needed to find a job that made good money and a partner that was stable?

The Good Girl Complex

From a young age, we're taught to disconnect from the things that bring us pleasure—especially as girls. Many women have shared stories with me of when they were young and were shamed for exploring their body. They were sent the message that you don't get to enjoy your body. That doing so is wrong and sinful and dirty: "Good girls don't do that." And so, like the good girls they so desperately wanted to be (because good girls are accepted and loved), they complied. They never realize that's why it's so hard for them to relax and enjoy sex decades later. Because they are running the program that good feelings in their body are bad and they are bad for enjoying them.

This is what I call the Good Girl Complex. As little girls, we're programmed to be good. Think about when your parents dropped you off somewhere. What's one of the last things they likely said to you, "Be good."

Maybe you've spoken those words to your own kids. And being good isn't a bad thing. But it becomes problematic when being good (according to society's standards) is the only thing that little girl focuses on for the rest of her life. When women are so used to being good, coloring inside the lines, dutifully checking everything off their to-do list, they put off pursuing things that light them up. They shun pleasure because they see it as a distraction from their pre-scripted role.

I want you to read that again. Pleasure is seen as a distraction: a *distraction*. And we avoid things that distract us because they derail us from our "greater" pursuits.

The Human Giver Syndrome

Author Kate Manne developed the theory that there are two classes of people: the human givers and the human beings. The human givers have a moral obligation to ensure the wellbeing and success of human beings. Human givers are expected to give of their time, talents, energies, and yes, even bodies, to fulfill the needs and desires of human beings. That means taking up less space physically, emotionally, sexually, and spiritually to avoid infringing on the human beings.

One of the messages for human givers is that pleasure isn't for them, it's for others. As human givers, we divorce ourselves from receiving and experiencing pleasure. "No, no, I don't need that" or "I'm good," are key phrases of human givers. Not just in the bedroom but in all facets of life. Human givers don't ask for anything. Why would they? They don't have needs. Their job is to attend to the needs of others all while being pretty, kind, patient, polite, and generous. Burnout from this Syndrome is usually what leads clients to contact me. They just can't do it anymore and they assume that something must be wrong with THEM, not the system that set them up to fail.

The Notebook **Dilemma**

As a young adult, one of my favorite movies was *The Notebook*. It reminded me of my own journey into marriage, though not nearly as dramatic. In high school and through my first year of college, I dated a wonderful guy. He was just like James Marsden's character, Lon. He was the "right" choice according to my parents. And while he checked all the boxes (loyal, smart, and financially secure), he didn't check any of my other "boxes," if you know what I mean. I just wasn't physically attracted to him.

Despite knowing this for the last year of our relationship, I suppressed those feelings. Why? Because it didn't feel safe to pursue pleasure and desire. Those were "worldly" things. Things that faded with time. True love, so I was told, was about commitment and shared values.

I decided one September day that I just couldn't do it anymore. I couldn't stay in a relationship where I had to pretend like I didn't want pleasure or desire. I decided that I was willing to forgo my security in hopes of finding someone someday who checked ALL my boxes. Ending that relationship was hard and heartbreaking. But it told the Universe that I was serious about wanting more. That I wasn't going to settle, and that pleasure was important to me (which I didn't actually know at the time, but looking back, I see it now).

Thankfully, I did find someone who checked all my boxes. Just like Noah and Allie, we had (and still do have) passion. Which doesn't always mean peace. But two decades later, I'd still choose my husband. I'd still trust my decision to pursue pleasure.

For those who don't make that choice, for those who settle, who don't realize why they're unhappy and dissatisfied, I understand why. Why would you pursue pleasure and desire when the messages you're receiving are packaged to us as follows:

- Pleasure is not for me, it's for you (the Human Giver Syndrome).
- Pleasure is a distraction (the Good Girl Complex).
- It's not safe to pursue pleasure and desire (*The Notebook* Dilemma).

Do any of these resonate with you? Because even after all the years of doing this work, I can still find elements in each of these that sound like me. That reflect my actions. Not nearly as often. No wonder I get blocked (cut off from my passion, sexuality, creativity, or desire to connect with others) professionally and personally. Maybe you do too.

Mind–Body Connection

One of the goals I have in working with my clients, regardless of the issues they come to me for, is reconciling the relationship they have with their bodies. I don't push for a client to go from hating their body to loving it overnight because, let's be honest, that's just not gonna happen. My goal is to help them realize that their body is a part of them. It is them, just as much as the mind is, so I encourage them to reconnect.

So often when it comes to solving "sex problems," practitioners and individuals focus on the mind. They ignore the body and its baggage. And this is why they don't end up with the long-term results they're wanting.

If you've felt betrayed by your body for any reason (e.g., infertility, weight issues, or illness), there can be resistance to reconnecting. One way to facilitate healing is by writing your body a letter. I know this sounds weird, but a lot of the stuff I say is, so let's just move right along. Your body won't understand the words, but she (yes, "she," not "it," or however you identify) will understand how the words make her *feel*.

Our bodies don't speak the same language our mind does. Our bodies understand emotion, sensation, and vibration. Those are nonverbal, and yet so often when we are in an unwanted state (i.e., anger), we tell ourselves (or we're told by others) to just "calm down." "Oh, you want me to just calm down? Well of course I will then," said no one ever. Our body responds to movement, music, and breath. No amount of logical reasoning will make a difference. This is why you can't just think your way to better sex or better whatever. You must also embody it.

Put on Your Shoes!

Have you ever seen the meme of the mom trying to get her kids to put their shoes on? The first image is of Mary Poppins telling the children politely and lovingly to please put on their shoes. And the next image is of a crazed person screaming at her kids to get their damn shoes on now. As Sheldon from *The Big Bang Theory* likes to say, "It's funny because it's true."

Our bodies work the same way. She will quietly whisper to us, "Hello? Hi, um, could you please pay attention to this ache, pain, or sensation? Thank you!" She's hoping, just like that mom, that we will listen. But as I'm sure you know, we rarely do. Instead, we push on because being productive is highly valued. This causes our bodies to get louder so then maybe we'll listen. We start to experience anxiety, migraines, irritable bowels, or heartburn. For many at this point, we start to listen because our performance, our ability to get things done, is now being affected. Sometimes we'll take a Tums or a Tylenol and push on through. We'll grumble about the setback but keep on keeping on.

Here's the thing—our bodies are relentless and WILL get our attention. Maybe not today or tomorrow, but our bodies will require a reckoning. Can you treat the symptoms? Of course, but if you don't address the root cause, then escalation will occur. Heart attacks, strokes, debilitating panic attacks, and autoimmune disease are usually the next level. I can't tell you how many patients my husband, a medical doctor, has treated who seemed healthy yet stroked out at 28 or had a medical condition that just didn't make any sense. Research is finally showing that untreated T/trauma is a significant contributor to our physical health.

All this is to say that you are not a machine. Your body is not a high-performing vehicle. We must care for the vessel we are in.

We only get one body. I hope that you will honor it with the love and care you deserve.

Caring for Your Body

You may be thinking, well that's a great idea, Courtney, caring for my body. But what does that even look like? Here are a few ways to explore, care, and honor your body:

- **Diet:** No, I don't mean go on *a* diet. I mean pay attention to your diet, the food you eat. Growing up, I heard things like, "Oh, don't eat that cause it's fattening" and "That's just wasted calories" and "That's bad for you." Food was never just food. It always carried a good or bad value. It took me years to undo all the messaging around food, and to be honest, sometimes those messages creep back in.

One of the best ways I've found to approach food is by asking this important question, "How will this help fuel my body?" It takes all the judgment out of the should-I-eat-this-or-not equation. It allows me to objectively evaluate how this food will or will not move me toward my health goals of being stronger and healthier. When I know something won't help fuel my body in a way that helps me feel stronger and healthier, say a margarita or a brownie, I don't shame myself for desiring it. Instead, I evaluate whether it's what I really want. And if the answer is that I do really want it, then I eat it. And I don't feel bad about it.

- **Movement:** I intentionally did not use the word *exercise* here because for many that's a triggering word. As a child, yes, a child, exercise was how I punished my body for eating too many things that weren't good for me. Despite being an athlete, I hated exercising. My dad used to tell me that the only way I could lose weight (I was about 12 years old at the time) was if I ran 5 miles every day. Guess what form of exercise I hated for most of my life? You guessed it —running.

You don't have to be a runner or a tennis player to move your body. You can dance, walk, or hike your way through life, perform yoga or pilates. I find that when I do things like run and hike in nature, I'm more connected to myself and to the greater world than when I'm pounding away in a gym on an elliptical machine, staring at a screen and praying the minutes will be up soon. Movement is a beautiful way to honor our bodies currently and challenge them to go farther or faster than we ever imagined.

- **Self-Touch:** Yes, I do mean that, but I also don't mean that. When was the last time you mindfully applied lotion to your legs? Or you soaked in a bubble bath and moved the water slowly on your skin? Or you lit a candle, put on your favorite Slow Jams and made yourself climax? Touching ourselves doesn't have to be an erotic act. It can just be a way we intentionally show care to ourselves.

One of my favorite movements in yoga is when I bring my knees to my chest while laying on my back and then wrap my arms around my legs. I give myself a big squeeze. I smile every time! It's nothing profound, but it's a small moment where I get to connect with my body and say, "thank you. I see you. I feel you. I love you." I rarely say or even think those words when I'm doing that squeeze, but that is what my smile is conveying to my body (remember, our bodies don't communicate via thoughts; they communicate via feelings and movement).

- **Clothing:** Ok, let's be real. When was the last time you bought yourself new underwear? Or a new bra? If you have underwear that has holes or are older than your 10-year old child, they have got. to. go. I'm serious! I'm not saying you need to run out to Victoria's Secret and go all crazy in the sexy, strappy lingerie section (although...), but let's get some quality undergarments for your lady parts.

Research shows that when we dress for success, we actually show up differently. We carry ourselves differently. We see ourselves differently—more positively. It's not about having the designer brand or spending hundreds of dollars on an item. It's about the quality of the garment and how you think about yourself (and thus feel about yourself) in the garment. But, Courtney, you may be thinking, I'd rather spend money on my kids or someone else. Fair point. But why is it that you are always the one that drops to the bottom of your list? Putting yourself first may feel selfish. What's wrong with being selfish? What's wrong with saying, you know what? I actually want to buy myself something, and that means that someone else is going to have to wait to get what they want. Being selfish doesn't make you a bad person, despite what our culture says. Being selfish allows you to elevate your needs and desires and go after what you want. Men have been doing this for centuries, and I don't see anyone accusing them of being selfish.

Self-Trust

"Ooh, um, I just don't know!" Lola exclaimed.

"That's ok," I reassured her. "Let's try another question. When you're at a new restaurant, is it hard for you to order something?"

"Yes," she laughed. "I never know what to order if I haven't been there before. I'll usually be able to narrow it down but then I don't know which one to pick so I'll just have my husband pick for me."

"Why do you have him pick for you?" I asked her.

"Because then if I don't like it, I can blame him," she said.

"Ok. Let's say your husband won't pick, and you are the one that has to pick. What then?"

Lola started biting her bottom lip, and considered the question. "Well, I guess, I don't know..."

I asked her, "What are you afraid of?"

"Picking the wrong one," she said.

"And do you see this anywhere else in your life?" I asked her.

She paused and began to nod her head, "Yes."

WE'RE TAUGHT at a young age to obey authority. This is necessary for the survival of our children. If kids just did whatever they wanted, they would get hurt or hurt others. We do this, establish authority and rules, because the part of the brain responsible for executive functioning (impulse control and decision making), doesn't fully form until the age of 24. Unfortunately, many adults don't remind children of their internal moral compass. Rather, a reliance on authority is born.

When studying child development, I was fascinated by Jean Piaget, the famous psychologist. He found that when equality and obedience to authority were in conflict, the child favored obeying the authoritative figure, disregarding their own moral compass. So if something felt wrong to the child, they would ignore that internal guidance system to obey authority. And when this choice gets rewarded (through praise or gifts), it creates a circuit in our brain: suppress the internal compass, seek external guidance and validation.

This is why it may be hard for you to make a mundane decision like what to order at a new restaurant. Or more important ones such as where to send your kid to school. Or who to marry or partner with. You likely don't have that authority figure directly in your life anymore. And you never learned how to trust that internal guidance system, your intuition. In fact, when you have trusted yourself in the past, maybe you were filled with regret because you felt like you made the wrong choice or made a bad decision. When this happens over time, it erodes your self-trust. And it prevents you from making decisions and taking action.

Intuition

During the spring of my senior year of high school, I came home after school and watched *Oprah* almost every day. There is one episode that I will never forget. Oprah's head of security, Gavin de Becker, was being interviewed on home safety or something boring. But then he started talking about how we easily ignore our intuition, especially as women. He shared a story of a woman who was riding in an elevator with a man who made her really uncomfortable. Instead of getting off for fear of making a scene, she ignored her gut telling her to run. That man followed her to her apartment and raped her.

I fully believe that our Intuition is hardwired into all of us. And yet so few of us tap into and tune into this incredible gift.

We don't know how, or we think it's weird or maybe we've never thought about this part of us.

Recently, my husband asked for my advice on what he should do in a particular situation. It was way out of my wheelhouse, so I asked him, "What does your gut tell you?" I reminded him that we all have the ability to figure out what to do. We just have to trust ourselves enough to do it.

Here's what I've seen in my work and personal life. There is a direct correlation between self-trust and self-worth. When both are low, that leads to indecision (i.e., the inability to confidently make decisions). The more you trust yourself, the more you value yourself. And when you trust and value yourself, you believe that there is no wrong decision.

We get so caught up in making the "right" decision, but I think it's important to note that it's not about being right. It's about being ok with yourself and the outcome if your decision doesn't work out the way you wanted. It's about having your own back. It's about seeing yourself as worthy and capable of facing anything. And when you do make that decision, it's about accepting it by recognizing how unproductive and draining and harmful it is to spin and spiral and second guess.

I'm asking you to tune into that small voice inside you. I'm asking you to consider how you've avoided trusting in yourself. How you've let yourself be silenced and become submissive and passive to pleasure. Not because you're weak or unintelligent. But because you didn't know there was another way. I hope you get to know the incredible woman that you are. The one who is capable of confident decisions. The one who is worthy of pleasure. The one who knows there is a life out there waiting for her.

Toolbox:

- Write your body (or a specific part of your body) a letter. Treat her (or however you identify your body) as a living entity. Feel the words you are writing to her. Play music or light a candle that sets the tone for how you want your body to feel as she receives the words you have for her.
- How am I caring for my body? Where is one area I could improve and show my body the care she deserves?
- Am I connected with my intuition? What's preventing me from listening to my body's intuition? How can I overcome this?
- Do I trust myself? What are two ways I can increase self-trust?

7

A LOOK UNDER THE HOOD

"What's wrong with me?" Nikki tearfully asked.

"What do you mean?" I asked.

"I mean, why does it take me so long to orgasm?" she blurted out. "And when I finally do orgasm, it's not from vaginal penetration. Like he has to go down on me or I have to use a vibrator during sex."

"Ah," I said, understanding what she meant. "Well, I want you to buckle up because what I'm about to tell you is going to rock your world."

Nikki looked at me hesitantly.

"I get your skepticism. I was skeptical too. But what society has taught us about sex, about what happens before, during, and after sex is just wrong," I explained.

"Have you ever watched a movie like the original *Top Gun* from the '80s?" I asked her.

"Oh, yeah," Nikki said.

"Ok, do you remember the sex scene?" I asked her.

"Yes, it was one of the best kissing scenes I remember. At least little girl Nikki thought it was amazing," she said with a laugh.

"Yes!" I exclaimed. "That's the point! When we're little, we're exposed to these examples of what we think erotic encounters should look like. We see these images and then believe that sex should be this synchronized coming together of two people who easily undress one another, passionately meet and of course, of course, climax together."

"Yes!" Nikki responded. "That's it. That's what I've been trying to create."

"You and most women I talk to," I told her.

THIS. IS. NOT. HOW. SEX. WORKS. Misinformation from the media has caused women to hate, doubt, and reject themselves sexually. They've believed that something must be wrong with them. They must be broken if their bodies don't respond or perform the way they see on TV.

I cannot emphasize how misled we have been about sex, especially as women. Everything that we've been taught about sex and sexuality is based on how a man's body works. Everyone has just assumed that a woman's body works the same way. So we have this standard of "normal" that women are holding themselves to, but in reality only about 20% of women respond the same way a man does.

What do I mean by that?

The media and cultural norms have perpetuated this idea that all men want sex all the time. We've reduced an entire section of our population to walking sex sticks. Do men, on average, have a higher sexual desire than women?

That's honestly hard for me to answer at this point because it hasn't been an even playing field. I want you to consider how boys are taught about masturbation versus how girls are. Usually, if a young girl is caught touching herself because it feels good when she does it, she is usually shamed with, "Don't do that! That's gross" or "wrong" or "yucky." When a young boy touches his penis, the reaction tends to be focused on the humor of his inappropriate erection. "Billy, stop touching your penis" is usually met with, "But, Mom! When I do, it gets bigger." Little boys are already advocating for their own pleasure. Little girls are not.

So back to the question, do men, on average, have higher sexual desire than women? Well, if girls received the same messages that boys do about sex, if women had the same freedoms that men did when it came to having multiple sexual partners (remember the slut shaming?), I'm not sure we'd really see a difference between genders and desire for sex.

Higher levels of testosterone do contribute to a higher desire for sex. But that is only one factor in a whole sexual system. If you have the hormonal help, it may be easier for you to experience arousal quicker. So we do see this in men, but only about 50% of men actually experience the spontaneous arousal that we see in the movies. Spontaneous arousal is unprompted and unexpected.

For example, a man may see a gorgeous woman walking down the street and suddenly he's turned on and ready to engage in sex. That's spontaneous arousal. Because he wasn't looking to be aroused, but as the French say, voila! something *spontaneously* triggered it. This type of arousal occurs in about 50% of men and fewer than 20% of women. So again, it's important to remember that this is not what we see in the media.

So how *do* most women, approximately 80%, react? Responsively. Basically, their body *responds* to things that are intentionally arousing. And unlike men who can be physically ready for sex in mere seconds, it can take women a bit longer to get aroused. I'm not talking orgasm. I'm talking about the body preparing for sex. This includes blood flowing to your vulva, nipples becoming erect, the vaginal canal lengthening, and vaginal lubrication.

I know this information can feel like a lot. I'm sharing percentages and dropping medical terminology. So before you give up on me, I want to remind you that the more in touch you are with your body, the more in touch you can become with your desire(s), sexually and otherwise. Because a woman who is connected to her desires is more able to experience pleasure in all facets of her life. And a woman connected to her passion, both inside and outside of the bedroom, is a powerful force.

"Men are Like Microwaves and Women are Like Toasters."

I don't remember where I heard this statement, but honestly I hated the expression, "men are like microwaves and women are like toasters," for a long time. Why? Because society values the microwaves over the toasters. We value someone who can produce and perform on the spot. Who can orgasm when they're "supposed" to. Nevertheless, this is a pretty accurate comparison of the arousal process. Most men (and some women) are like microwaves—they can heat up pretty quickly, whereas a toaster (most women) can take several minutes to get fired up.

Once women are in this arousal stage, many people don't realize that moving to the climax can take them 10 to 20 minutes. Do you know how long most men last (before they ejaculate) during intercourse? Three to seven minutes. That's a 7 to 17-minute discrepancy! No wonder so many women are sexually unsatisfied. But the bigger issue I see is the sense of brokenness these women feel. Instead of understanding the biological process, they assume there must be something wrong with them because it takes longer than 3 to 7 minutes for them to orgasm. I know I did. When my body didn't respond the way I had seen in the movies, when I didn't climax simultaneously with my spouse, I blamed myself. "What am I doing wrong?" morphed into "What was wrong with me?" And sadly, no one was there to share this information with me. Instead, I was surrounded by other women just as frustrated and full of shame as I was.

Unfortunately, most men are unaware of this biological reality as well. So they too get frustrated. They internalize the inability to sexually "satisfy" their female partner. They may even shame their partner when she doesn't climax when they do. Because if their education is anything like that of most Americans, what you see modeled in the movies (looking at you, porn industry), leads one to believe that orgasming simultaneously IS the norm. I mean, can you think of a film or show when it shows the woman orgasming after the man? I can't either.

You're not broken. The world we live in and the messages we receive are. I truly believe that as soon as we begin to understand how our bodies respond and the impact cultural messaging has on us, we can take control of our sexual functioning.

Brakes and Gas

Researchers have used numerous models over the years to try and explain the female sexual response cycle. One of my favorite models, because I'm nerdy like that, is the dual control model of sexual response by Dr. John Bancroft and Dr. Erick Janssen. In a Kinsey Institute Report, they explain that "The Dual Control Model reflects the idea that sexual response in individuals is the product of a balance between excitatory and inhibitory processes." What does that mean?

I want you to imagine a car. Now imagine you're sitting in the driver's seat. At your feet are a gas pedal and brake pedal. The accelerator or the excitatory process is the gas pedal. This is your body responding to any sexual information relevant in your environment—everything you see, hear, touch, smell, taste, or imagine that your brain assigns as sexually significant. It then sends the "turn on" signal (i.e., it pushes the gas pedal down).

At the same time, the inhibitory or brake pedal is noticing all the reasons *not* to be turned on right now. It also uses the same information from your environment—everything you see, hear, smell, touch, taste or imagine that's a potential threat—and it sends a signal that says "turn off" (i.e., pump the brake). So, arousal is not just the process of turning on the ons, it's also turning off the offs.

Have you ever pushed the brake and the gas pedals at the same time? What happens? Well, the engine revs but you don't go anywhere because the brake is more powerful than the accelerator. Let me repeat that—the brake, what turns you off, is way more powerful than the gas, what turns you on. So you can be at the most romantic resort in Jamaica with your sweetie, with the kids at home in Minnesota, and you may still not be able to "get in the mood," because that brake, the stimulus turning you off, will always win.

When I work with clients, one of the things we do is identify their gas pedal (turn-ons) as well as their brake pedals (turn-offs). This is where most clinicians miss the boat. They're super focused on the gas pedal. "Go buy some lingerie, send the kids to grandma's, bust out the sex toys—you'll be fine!" So when the woman does this and there still is a disconnect, they tell her to push harder on the gas pedal. She's made to feel even more stigmatized for her inability to figure it out and get it together. So what does she do? She fakes it. She suppresses her frustration, ignores the guilt, and puts on a good show for her partner. All the while, she can't wait for them to be done so she can go back to doing something she actually wants to do.

I'm here to tell you that there is nothing wrong with you if you haven't figured out why you can't just sit back, relax, and enjoy the ride. Because I'm sure you've tried that. I'm sure you've tried to take a bath before you get busy. I'm sure you've tried drinking a glass of wine or three to just de-stress. Maybe you've even flipped through the *Kama Sutra* in hopes of finding that magical position. Can all of these be helpful resources (well, maybe not the three glasses of wine)? Sure, but I want to go deeper by helping you identify why that may be difficult to do.

In the last chapter we talked about The Good Girl Complex, Human Giver Syndrome, and *The Notebook* Dilemma. If you identify with ANY of these, then you probably have a good idea what's pushing down your brake pedal. And it's important to know that some women just have a more sensitive brake than others. You may have a friend who grew up in the same purity culture you did, but who is able to enjoy sex more easily than you are. That doesn't mean there's something wrong with you. It means you push down more easily on your brakes or need a lot more umph to get the gas going.

When I talk to women about why it's hard for them to enjoy sex, here are some of the things they say:

- "It's hard to relax when I know there's a sink full of dishes (or laundry or bills...) waiting for me when we're done."
- "I'm afraid the kids will hear us or walk in on us."
- "I'm so tired. I'd rather sleep."
- "I don't want another baby."
- "I don't know how to switch from mommy mode to wife mode."

I could go on (and I'm sure you've got some of your own). All of these are rooted in one of those concepts from the last chapter.

Sadly, you don't win anything if you identify with all three categories. But you do gain awareness of where your issues are rooted. And self-awareness is step number one.

Why?

Growing up in the church, I heard the parable of the house built on the sand a lot. The parable is found in the Gospel of Matthew, Chapter 7. Here, Jesus instructs his audience to put into practice what they are learning. He compares this to building your house on a rock instead of being foolish (by not applying Jesus' teachings) and building it on the sand. Because sand is unstable. A house built on the sand will not sustain the storms. As I touched on in the very beginning of this book, your Why is your foundation.

One of the forms I ask new clients to fill out is called "Your Why." It's a short one-pager with a couple questions on it. The first question I ask is: *Who are you doing this for?*

If the client answers that they are doing it for anyone other than themselves, I discuss this at the beginning of our first session. I want to acknowledge that if you've struggled with doing anything for yourself, it can feel weird to shyly raise your hand and say, "I'm doing this for me."

As women, we've been conditioned to put the needs of others before our own. We've been taught that being selfish is one of the worst things we could be called. So yes, putting your own needs and desires first, showing up for yourself, can feel odd and a bit uncomfortable. I'm here to tell you to sit with those feelings and do it anyway.

"I NOTICED that you put you were doing this for your spouse on the 'Your Why' form," I said to Barb.

Barb smiled proudly and confidently stated, "Yes! I am. I'm doing this so we can have a better sex life."

"I think that's a great goal. I'm curious why you didn't include that you were doing all this work, because what we're doing is not easy, for yourself," I said.

Barb scrunched her face a little and looked at me confused. "Why would I be doing this for me? I'd be fine with never having sex again. And as you said, it's a lot of work, so no, I'm not doing this for me."

"Ok!" I responded enthusiastically. "That is exactly the kind of honesty I want here. The problem with doing things that others want us to do is that the results don't last. For example, have you ever tried picking up a sport or hobby or even tried losing weight because of something someone said to you?"

Barb nodded, "Yes. My spouse really wanted me to play pickleball and I hated it. So I signed up for lessons thinking that would make them happy. Showing them that I'm trying for them."

I smiled, knowing the answer to the question I was about to ask, "How's your pickleball game?"

Barb huffed and stated, "I don't play pickleball anymore."

I nodded my head, "Exactly."

WHEN WE DO things for others that we really don't want to do, but feel like we should do, we create a little box labeled Resentment inside of us. Usually, we can white knuckle through these unwanted tasks others require of us. However, over time, our willpower fades. We reflect on the progress we have made but feel guilty about not making a true change, ultimately abandoning the original cause.

Maybe you picked up this book for your partner. Maybe you

thought you'd learn a thing or two on how to keep them satisfied or appease them more frequently.

Can I ask you to do something really important right now? Well, I'm going to, but I wanted to get your consent first. Can you commit to reading every word from here on out, for YOU? Can you choose, in this space we have left together, to put yourself, your needs, your questions and concerns first? Because I could give you all the insight into your body and societal expectations and communication, but if you're doing this for anyone other than yourself, it won't matter.

I want you to see that you matter. You matter enough to read this book for you. Because you are worthy of good and amazing things, but you can't experience them until you choose yourself first.

It's Not Their Job

I grew up with the notion that your other half was out there somewhere waiting to be found. The church didn't qualify this as having a soulmate, but popular culture did. And what an appealing message it is: you aren't "this" (whatever this is) because you're not whole. You're incomplete until you find the one and only that allows everything to magically fall into place. Then you'll be successful and fulfilled. And live happily ever after.

Spoiler alert: that's not only untrue, it's harmful. The belief that single people are incomplete as they are is just, well, insulting. And the idea that it's your partner's responsibility to somehow complete you is problematic. As much as I'd love to discuss the implications of this belief, I will narrow my focus to how this affects women sexually.

If you're not encouraged to understand your body by exploring it and you're told that when you grow up and get married, you will have amazing sex because you saved yourself for your husband (looking at you, purity culture), then of course, you'd expect your spouse to be one amazing lover. To know exactly how to please you. This mentality places you at the disposal of your partner and their ability to arouse you.

But isn't that what we're supposed to do as sexual partners? Arouse and please each other? Short answer—no. Longer answer—it's not our partner's responsibility to turn us on or give us pleasure. The responsibility is ours. To identify what turns us on. To determine what feels good and what doesn't. And then to communicate those insights to our partner so they can partake in the pleasure with us. They may not physically feel the pleasure you do when they hit that one spot you love, but they do experience pleasure knowing they are able to do that for you.

Too often I see women who show up to sexy time as passive participants. They're filled with sentiments such as "they're not doing it the way I like it," but we're too scared to tell our partners that truth. So we hope and pray they'll figure out that we've stopped moaning or our breathing has slowed down all the while we're losing momentum and just want this act to be over. Our partners aren't mind readers. It's unfair of us to expect them to know what we want and how we want it.

When we claim responsibility and take ownership of our arousal and pleasure, we show up to sex differently. Heck, we show up to life differently. We are more likely to advocate for our needs. We are more confident in how we carry ourselves. We take better care of our minds and bodies because we know we are sacred, sexual vessels worthy of pleasure.

Toolbox:

- How can I give myself grace knowing what I know now about arousal and orgasm?
- What are the things that push my gas? What are the things that push my brake?
- Why am I doing this for me?
- How have I been expecting my partner to arouse me? How can I take ownership of my own arousal?

8

SEXUAL ENERGY

If there was a recipe for successful sexual energy, I promise you it would've been created, copyrighted, and sold out a million times over. But there isn't. There is no one way. And part of your journey in this life is to find your way. In this case, your way back to your sacred sexual energy. Because it's always been there. You didn't lose it. You suppressed it for a thousand reasons.

Sadly, we've become divorced from our senses. Our senses are powerful. They're the gateway to our bodies. They are the mind–body bridge. Sensual living is a portal for creating and accessing your sexual energy. We were created to experience the world through our senses. And yet when was the last time you ate your food without utensils? When was the last time you actually stopped to smell the roses or any kind of flower? The message, again from the patriarchy, is that you can't trust your body. You can't give into your desires.

This is why so many of the women I talk to have no idea what they want. Not just out of life but also what THEY want for dinner. Or what they want to do for fun. They've accepted that deflecting to others and putting everyone else's needs before their own is virtuous. I'm not talking about being self-centered or obstinate. I'm talking about believing that you're not entitled to define for yourself how you want to spend your time and how you get to experience this life.

My Wake-Up Call

It was the summer of 2017. I woke up at 3:00 a.m. itching like crazy. "Not another thing," I thought to myself as I limped out of bed and into the bathroom. I turned on the light and was shocked to see bumpy red hives all over my chest. Normally, I would wake up my husband and ask him what to do (the benefits of being married to a physician). But my husband was working in another state and had poor cell phone service. So I scoured our bathroom shelves looking for something, anything that would make the itching stop. I'm pretty sure I took some expired Benadryl, but I was so desperate, I didn't care.

And really, that desperation was what propelled me to understand how my energy was affecting my physical body. At the time, I had no idea that there was a connection or what the energetic body even was.

The Benadryl I took gave me relief for a few days. But the hives came back. I went to my doctor. He ran some tests, and everything came back normal. If I wasn't having an allergic reaction, then what was going on? I had no idea, but I started searching for answers.

A friend told me that stress could be causing my hives.

"Stress?" I laughed. "What could I be stressed about?"

"Well," she said cautiously, "your dad died a few months ago. Then your family dog died 2 months after that. And your husband is gone all summer working. What do you mean, what could you be stressed about?"

"I just thought those are things that happen. I dealt with them and then moved on," I said callously.

"Apparently you haven't," she told me lovingly. "Your body is trying to get you to pay attention."

"To what?" I asked her.

"I don't know," she said. "That's something you have to figure out. But you shouldn't do it alone. Work with a professional. Have you tried acupuncture?"

"Where they stick needles in you?" I asked.

"Yes," she said. "But it's more than that. You should check it out."

I was so desperate to feel better that I did check it out. And it completely changed my life.

OUR ENERGETIC BODY serves as an intermediary between our physical body and our psychological self. Here's one way to consider the energetic body. Have you ever felt a burst of passion or a potent charge of emotion surge inside you? Have you ever been attracted to someone else? How can you really tell? Or here's a better question—what did you feel? It's hard to describe, right? But that's the energetic body's feeling of being activated. That is what you're tuning into though you may have never realized it before.

What about this—have you ever walked into a room and noticed that it just felt weird? Or even said to yourself, "the energy just feels off in here?" Part of what you're picking up on is the energy of the people in the room. You can't see it with your own eyes, but you can sense it. Or maybe you've met someone, and all of your friends love them. Yet, there's just something about them you can't quite identify, so you just aren't a fan? You're picking up on their energy (which is expressed through their energetic body).

Different philosophies categorize these energy bodies in different ways. The most popular system, found in the Hatha Yoga tradition, is the chakra system. The chakra system is similar to a spiritual nervous system. The most common system (at least in the West) specifies seven chakras that run along (not in) a person's spine. Each chakra (translated as "wheel" in Sanskrit) is believed to hold thoughts, feelings, and memories related to specific areas of our life. When we tap into a chakra (which anyone can do), we are able to connect with a part of the energetic body. Just like our physical body, our energetic body can get stuck or blocked. Just like we can show symptoms from a virus or cold in our physical body, we can show symptoms of overactive or underactive chakras in our energetic one.

The chakra system has an uncanny correlation to our endocrine system, which is considered to be the body's master command center when it comes to emotions and bodily functions. The locations and functions of the glands or organ directly relate to the location of the Chakra. For example, the sacral chakra, located in the pelvis region, right below the naval, is linked to the reproductive organs. The sacral chakra, just like the reproductive organs, is responsible for pleasure, creation, and birth.

I've been trained in Usui Reiki, an energy healing practice that works with the chakra system. When I saw I couldn't find answers in Western medicine (or Western practices) alone, I searched for more. And that led me to acupuncture and Reiki. These modalities have allowed me to view the person as more than just a brain. Eastern philosophies honor the mind and body by affirming their connection, not discounting it. I still very much believe in Western, evidence-based medicine. And I embrace esoteric approaches, holding both models as options and outlooks for healing the mind, body, and spirit.

Our energy body has always been a part of us, though most

of us were never aware that it existed. One of my goals in writing this is for you to have an increased awareness about all parts of your body, including this one. Your chakras have been active your entire life, though they develop as we do. Our life force resides in each of the chakras. Each center holds a different purpose and embodies a part of us unlike the others, yet still integral to our overall system.

When your chakras are healthy and balanced, life feels uncomplicated. It flows. Things move in a way that makes sense on an instinctual level. It doesn't mean that you don't face hardship. It's just that when you do, you know that you will come out stronger because of it. Your energy body is always speaking to you.

Each chakra has its own location and purpose. We're not going to dive into all of them; instead, we'll focus on the sacral chakra, which is the energy center for passion and sensuality. It's the part of you that lights up when your lips meet those of the person you've been longing for. Or when you feel the words of a moving song. Or when you see the sky painted in reds, oranges and purples on a summer night. Or when you hold a life you created in your arms for the first time.

Located in the pelvic region and in the traditional female womb space is your sacral chakra. This second chakra is where women's energetic bodies are anchored. In many traditions, the color representing the sacral chakra is orange; its symbol is an orange six-petaled flower. Qualities most often associated here include sexuality, feminine power, fluidity, and adaptability. It's important to acknowledge that our sacral chakra, this part of our body, is not just about sex. I find it fascinating and encouraging that the same place that houses our sexuality is the same one that our creativity and passion call home. You don't have to have given birth to a human to have birthed something inspiring and creative. This place exists in every person and is our birthright. The place that houses our sexual energy, that has the power to create life (literally and metaphorically), exists in our sacral chakra.

What many don't realize is that the sacral chakra is also responsible for our creativity, inspiration, desires, and passions. These are qualities that enhance and facilitate enjoyment in our lives. If we didn't have inspiration, we would be without art and music. Life would merely be cerebral. Inspiration is what connects us to our own humanity and our fellow humans.

Living in Color

Our chakras are our life force energy. They allow us to connect with ourselves and others in different ways. When we tap into these chakras it's almost like going from living in black and white to finally living in full color.

I'm reminded of the late '90s movie, *Pleasantville*, where modern day siblings (Reese Witherspoon and Toby McGuire) are sucked into the television and transported into the brother's favorite television show, *Pleasantville*, which centers on an idyllic 1950s family. When the characters arrive, they are shocked that everything remains in black and white, including themselves. Eventually the siblings inspire the other characters to break free from both internal and external repression. This is ultimately symbolized by a character turning into color. I see our sacral chakra the same way. Our body can carry us from activity to task to sleep to shower. But unless we allow ourselves the opportunity to embody these experiences, we are merely robots being run by our subconscious mind (similar to a computer running a program in the background).

When our sacral chakra is blocked, we get stuck emotionally, physically, and sexually. Life doesn't move with ease and flow. It feels more like walking knee-deep in mud. Everything resists.

And when we're constantly facing resistance and struggle, we want to check out. Because life's not very fun so we want to find a way to escape.

Let me give you an example. Have you ever put your kids (or someone's kids) to bed before? When you do this night after night after night, it can feel a bit draining. You put them in the bath. You read the story. And you keep checking your watch to see when this will be over so you can just go sit down and not have anybody bother you. When things don't go as planned ("just ONE more story, Mommy, please!"), you think, "This is taking too long!" (I wonder where else we say this…).

Now, imagine the same scenario but this time, you're present. You're intentional. As they step out of the bathtub, you smell their little, clean heads as you dry them off. You pick a story that you love doing different voices of all the characters. You experience bedtime *with* your kiddos. You feel the love and connection. You enjoy this time with them. You honor the power of the present moment and fully allow it to envelop you. This is an embodied experience.

When we are receptive to connecting with our partner and their body, we are saying, "I'm here. I'm here for all of it. I want to feel and experience this moment." When we are open to finding joy in the little things, in ourselves, we can receive and experience pleasure more easily.

Please remember that nourishing your passion and your sacral chakra energy isn't yet another thing you have to add to your to-do list. It's really about tuning into this sacred part of you.

One of the things I really want every reader to walk away from this book knowing is that they are the ones who hold the key to their own healing. You may not have the medicine or know how to administer it, but you do know when something is off and when you've lost your way. Understanding all the parts of us gives us power in coming home to ourselves. In connecting back to our sacred sexual energy.

The more connected you are to your sexual energy, the more possibilities there are. Not from out there. But from in here. In *you*. And as you expand in possibility so does your world. This is an awakening. And as you awaken, you are given the opportunity to align your beliefs, relationships, and energy in a way that honors this new connection with yourself.

Let Me Clear My Throat

There's one more energy center that's vital to our journey. Our ability to speak clearly, to listen intently, is related to our throat chakra. This is located at our throat and is often referred to as the communication chakra. I find it interesting that this energy center relies on vibration, movement, and thought because these elements are directly connected to how our bodies process experiences.

AYA SHOWED up one session and was complaining about her neck and shoulders bothering her. Before we began our session, I asked her if she was familiar with the energetic body.

"Not really," Aya responded.

"That's ok," I told her. "Most people aren't. Sometimes it's easier to understand the energetic body when we can identify where energy is being blocked, kind of like a traffic jam. I want you to imagine that there's a highway, running from the top of your head all the way to the base of your spine. Now, imagine that there are traffic circles at certain points along this highway. Sometimes there are backups or full-on accidents at these points. And when this happens, we can feel those backups or blocks or accidents in our body as sensations like tightness or soreness or in our emotions like sadness, anxiety, depression, anger. Does that make sense?"

"Yes," she said curiously.

"Ok, so those sensations or feelings we get in our body are messages. It's our body's way of speaking to us, trying to get our attention," I explained.

"What's my tight neck and sore shoulders trying to tell me then?" Aya asked with a laugh.

I smiled and asked her "Well, are you struggling with speaking up or speaking your truth lately? Or are you having a hard time really listening to others?"

She nodded her head and said, "Funny you should ask me that. My mother-in-law is in town, and I get so frustrated with all her little comments about my parenting. It drives me crazy! But I can't say anything because I have to keep the peace."

"Well your body doesn't like that, that you feel like you can't speak up. It's unsettling and that is causing a block in your throat chakra," I explained while pointing to my throat. "Remember those traffic circles I was telling you about? Well one of those roundabouts is located right here, at your throat. And those traffic circles are called chakras. This is your throat chakra."

"Interesting," she said.

I explained, "Our energetic body is a field of incredible information that surrounds our physical body. It also processes experiences, events, and other energy, just like our brain and body do. In this case, you don't feel comfortable or confident enough to speak up to your mother-in-law. But those feelings of frustration, anger, and resentment don't magically go away just because you don't know how to deal with them. They get stuck in the body; in this case, in your neck and shoulders."

"Wow," she said. "I never realized that."

"You're not alone," I said. "I didn't either for a long time."

．　．　．

WHEN YOUR THROAT chakra is clear, you can communicate effectively and with ease. Individuals notice that they can listen as well as express their feelings without difficulty. A balanced throat chakra also allows us to understand the meaning beyond or behind words. It is also connected to our writing and musical abilities. If you've ever struggled with writer's block or have difficulty conveying information to someone, you could have a blocked throat chakra. Balancing this part of you gives you the power to speak up and share your truth with the world.

I have two master's degrees. One in sexuality education and one in mental health counseling. I don't share this to toot my own horn. I share this because in both of those programs, I never learned about the energetic body. Everything I've been taught in traditional, formal education was focused on the neck up. Ok, sure we learned about biology in one of my programs, but 95% of the rest of the stuff I learned was centered on the brain. Now, the brain is obviously an important player in all of this. But it's not the only one. There's a whole other world out there, and it exists in and slightly above our skin.

The Power of Presence

So how do you connect with your body? How do you start to embody your emotions so you can align your beliefs, relationships, and energy? By being present. It's a simple concept, but definitely a difficult process. Our brains spend so much time living in the past and trying to predict and control the future. Rarely are we present. And as I mentioned earlier, if we don't feel safe in our bodies, disconnection from the present is a coping mechanism.

So how can we be present? One powerful way is through

grounding. Grounding, just like an electrical current, involves plugging into or anchoring into a larger force. You don't have to believe in a specific spirituality or religion to ground. If you do have a spiritual practice—awesome, let's incorporate that. Just know that you can approach grounding in so many ways.

The most important element is connecting to the Earth. Connecting to, well, the ground beneath you. Literally. Walk in the grass barefoot. Get your hands in the dirt by gardening or picking flowers. Touch the trees on a nature walk. And pay attention to the sensations. Feel the ground meeting you, holding you in your current space.

You can even just stand. Stand still. Close your eyes and affirm your own authority over yourself. Summon the strength in your legs. See that you are safe, strong, and protected in this moment. Because it's all about this moment. Not ruminating on the past, not trying to predict the future.

When you do this regularly, you balance this chakra. You encourage your mind to be present fully in your body. And as you are able to be present, to feel safe, and be in your body, the foundation for self-trust and self-love is laid.

Self-love is a bit of a buzzword. What I'll say about self-love here is that you can't hate yourself into change. Trust me, I've tried. And so have thousands of the women (and men) I've worked with. Love is the only true catalyst of change.

When we love ourselves and our bodies, shame and self-doubt dissipate. It doesn't happen overnight, which is why it's so important to stay consistent. You will get pushback from your brain. Your brain doesn't like change. Because change is scary and unpredictable. That's why it's important to move the needle slightly at first. Gradual change leads to change that lasts.

Toolbox:

- How do I feel about the energetic body and this hidden power?
- What is one way I will intentionally connect with my sacral chakra?
- What are ways my sacral chakra could be blocked?
- How do I feel about self-love? Am I currently loving myself to change or hating myself for where I am?

PART III

MOVING FORWARD

I never understood why I had to learn about history in school. It's so boring, I thought. We can't change the past, so why are we studying it? Ugh. I see this approach with clients sometimes. They are hesitant to discuss things from their past: "I can't change what happened to me, Courtney, so what's the point in talking about it? It's hard and it hurts." The thing is, they're not wrong. It is hard to talk about because that pain still feels very real.

Here is what I've realized about the past—it never really goes away. Our bodies don't process time the same way our minds do. So if we don't acknowledge what has happened to us, if we don't release that which is trapped within us, it will not go away just because we want to move on. When we understand the past, when we examine how it has impacted us, and when we learn that incredibly important lesson (which is different for everyone), then we can create a future that is filled with freedom. And from this place of freedom, we can transform our own lives. And a woman who has that power to transform her life, that is a woman who can transform the world.

9

MODALITIES

"So, like how does this work?" Jay asked me.

"How does what work?" I asked him.

"This," he said, motioning to the space between himself and me.

"Oh," I stated, realizing what he was asking. "Well, there are lots of ways we could do this," I say, mirroring his previous motions. "There are actually more than 50 different approaches to therapy—50! If you've never been to a therapist's office before, maybe you have a mental image of someone lying on a couch, talking away while the clinician silently jots down notes. Or maybe you've seen some reality shows where the therapist and client have more of a conversation that's guided by the therapist."

"Oh, yeah," he said. "I've seen both of those kinds."

"The way I approach this is a combination of several methods. When I was in graduate school, the gold standard of therapy was cognitive-behavioral therapy (CBT). This is the belief that our thoughts, feelings, and behaviors are all connected. If you want to change one of those elements, say your behavior, then you need to change how you think and feel.

Want to change how you feel? Change how you behave and think."

He nodded and said, "Yeah, ok. That makes sense."

"So then why don't we just fix what doesn't work and easily resolve our issue?" I asked him.

He tilted his head, considering my question. "Hmm. Yeah, I don't know. I mean, it sounds so easy. Is it that easy?"

"Well," I began, "I used to think so, yes. I honestly believed that if you wanted to change your behavior, you had to change your thoughts. Everything really started with the thoughts. But the more I started to understand the brain, the less confident I was in this one approach to helping people."

"So what's the answer?" he asked me.

I laughed a little at his question because I too had wondered that. If there was a problem, that meant there had to be a solution, right? But what if the problem was actually the problem? Meaning, what if the way we looked at our brains, our minds, was problematic? That would explain why these so-called simple solutions were falling short. Why we couldn't just think our way to better sex or smaller bodies.

"So there's this way of looking at how our mind works. It's gonna sound a little out there, so stay with me, ok?" I asked my client.

"We're this far already," he jokingly said, "so whatcha got?"

"Have you ever heard of Cybil? The woman with multiple personalities," I asked him.

"Yes," he said.

I took a deep breath in and began, "Most mental health practitioners look at the mind as one unit. And anything that is fragmented is abnormal or pathological, like Cybil was. But what if the brain were actually multiple on its own? I know that sounds, well, crazy. So, let's break it down. Have you ever felt like a part of you wanted to do one thing but then another part of you wanted to do another? What if those parts were actually separate parts inside you?"

"Yeah," he responded, "I've had that with a lot of things actually. I guess I never considered that they could be separate parts."

I continued, "Most people haven't. In fact, most of us don't because of the association with multiple personalities," I told him. "I love this way of looking at the mind because it doesn't stigmatize or pathologize (diagnose someone as having something wrong with them). Instead, part of the mind is trying to protect us from something because of a big 'T' or little 't' trauma or experience from the past. That part isn't trying to hurt us or make our lives more difficult. I know that's what it feels like it's doing! But it's just trying to protect us from pain."

"Yeah, I never thought about it like that," he said.

I said, "I find that it's an incredibly compassionate way to look at our behaviors. And that's really what I want for you, Jay, and all my clients. To increase the compassion and understanding you have for what you do and who you are."

So LET's apply this approach to sex. Maybe you struggle with desire. And maybe you've tried to ease up on the things that turn you off (remember the chapter on brakes and gas?). But you still find yourself disconnected or easily distracted or just not in the mood. Still, a part of you wants to connect with your partner. That part is the Self. The core of who you are. The undamaged essence that defines you. In Internal Family Systems, the model that explains all of this, the Self is best described with the 8 Cs.

When an individual is

- Calm
- Curious

- Creative
- Courageous
- Connected
- Compassionate
- Confident
- And has clarity,

they are in their true Self state. And when they're in this state, they are able to heal themselves. When the Self has the five Ps

- Presence
- Persistence
- Playfulness
- Patience
- Perspective

it allows us to see our relationships and experiences differently, which is a powerful way to heal our past. The eight Cs and five Ps aren't an exhaustive checklist. You don't need every quality to experience relief or healing. Rather, it's a guide to what is possible and what lies within each of us.

Sometimes our Self gets crowded out by parts that don't trust the Self or don't know about it because our Self hasn't been able to run things. Let's look at Maya's situation.

"Why can't I figure this out?" Maya said to me.

"Figure what out?" I asked her.

"This," she said, motioning toward her body. "Like I bought the lingerie. I even let my husband buy me a sex toy. And it helped for like a month. But I just feel like I'm back to where I started."

"And feeling guilty about being back there?" I asked her.

"Yes!" she exclaimed. "Like can this ever be fixed?"

"Of course," I told her honestly. "But it's not a quick fix. There's a reason part of you or parts of you aren't on board with matching your husband's enthusiasm for sex."

"Parts of me?" she asked.

"Yes," I began. "So, let's look at your current situation. Would you say that part of you really desires to be sexual with your husband?"

"Yes," she stated.

"But there's also a part of you that's disengaged?" I asked.

"Yes, that part always seems to win out," she said.

"And maybe there's another part of you that wants to be desired or wooed or whatever?" I asked.

"Absolutely," she said.

"What if those different parts of you were actually parts inside you. Kind of like a family. Everyone has different needs and different agendas but they're all working together for the most part. Or they at least share some common goals," I explained.

"Sure, I get that," Maya stated.

"Let's do an exercise," I told her. "I want you to think of an image, word, feeling, or thought that you have about sex."

Maya took in a deep breath and said, "Ok, let me think of one..."

"No rush," I told her.

"Ok, got one. I have an image of my husband moving next to me after we get into bed together. It's his way of initiating sex," she said.

"Great. Now I want you to close your eyes and take a couple deep breaths. And just settle into your body," I told her. I wait for her to relax and then say, "I want you to notice whether you can feel that image in, on, or around your body."

Within seconds Maya stated, "I feel like a knot in my stomach."

"Ok, that's normal," I reassured her. "Now, how do you feel toward it? Toward that knot in your stomach?"

Maya paused and answered, "Sad. I feel sad."

"Ok," I told her. "That's another part of you. Just ask that part to step aside for now. Thank it for wanting to protect you and ask whether it will let you focus on that knot in your stomach. Tell it that you want to help that knot in your stomach."

"Ok..." she said hesitantly.

I wait a few moments and checked back in. "How do you feel toward that knot in your stomach now?"

"I don't feel it as much," Maya said in a surprised tone. "That's weird. It's like it went away or something."

"That's good. So let's ask the knot in the stomach what it wants you to know," I told her.

"Like I just say that to the knot in my stomach?" she asked.

"Yep, just talk to it like you would a person," I instructed her.

"Ok..." she agreed.

I waited a little bit and checked in, "Did it respond?"

Maya laughed a little, "Actually, it did. It said, 'you can't trust others,' which surprised me."

"Can you ask it whether there's anything it wants to show you?" I told her.

Maya took a moment and then stated, "It's showing me a time when I was a little girl. I used my birthday money to buy my friends some friendship bracelets. And then I gave them the bracelets and they didn't really care."

"How did that little girl feel?" I asked her.

She said, "Sad. Rejected. But that little girl just kept doing things like that. She'd give up her lunch or even clothes to friends in hopes that they would accept her and include her," she explained.

"What if that's the part that is afraid of being fully present and vulnerable during sex? That little girl inside you is afraid of being rejected or used? So this part has found a way to protect you from having to feel those feelings."

Tears began to run down her face. "How..." she begins to say. "How did I never see this connection?"

"Because it's a different way of looking at our minds," I explained to her. "Because most people aren't equipped to make these kinds of connections. But you're here now, and that's what matters."

THIS IS an example of doing Parts Work. It's how I help individuals understand the connection between early (often traumatic) experiences and conditioning and their current struggles. It's how clients bridge the gap between their minds and bodies. And it's one of the most effective and powerful tools I've used in all my years of working in this field.

A stale sex life is always a symptom of a larger issue. When clients come to me and want help in this area of their life, they're usually unaware that there's a larger issue at play. Parts Work allows me the opportunity to identify what those larger issues are.

Our minds are incredibly powerful. Regardless of what theory you subscribe to, the mind's number one objective is to keep you safe. That means anything that threatens your safety, whether that's physical, emotional, financial, spiritual, or sexual, will be registered as a threat. And threats are to be avoided at all costs. One way our mind does this is by developing beliefs about the world.

Let's go back to Maya's situation. At a young age, she was rejected by her friends. Even after offering them a gift, they still didn't really seem to accept her. Our brains are meaning-making machines, so even if Maya's friends weren't trying to be hurtful or rude, her brain still made it mean that they were. And rude and hurtful people are registered as a threat in our brain. Maya, of course, was unaware that this was happening. But a seed was planted.

As a protective mechanism, parts of Maya's brain developed beliefs like, "others can't be trusted" and "you're not good enough" and "you're not worthy." Left unchecked, these seeds grew into a full-blown forest. The intention of these parts isn't to prevent Maya from having a great sex life or from connecting with her husband. The intention is to protect that little girl who was hurt all those years ago.

To heal yourself now, you have to heal that part of you that was hurt so long ago. To do that, you have to walk into the woods you've created.

Another way our mind protects us is by automating. Our brain loves to preserve energy, and what better way to do this than by going on autopilot. Unfortunately, when our brains are left unchecked, we can spend about 95% of our life operating on the unconscious level (not on the conscious, intentional level).

Think about your own routines. How different is each day from the next? I'm talking about minor movements like reaching for your phone first thing in the morning, then getting up and going to the bathroom. Then moving into the morning coffee, dropping off kids, going to work, driving home, making meals, putting kids to bed, doing the dishes...How much of your day is actually that different from the rest? It's predictable and routine. Which is not a bad thing. The problem is when these routines allow us to check out. When something is automated, you don't have to be present to make it happen. You can set and go. And our minds do. So when you're in bed with someone you love and want to connect, guess what your mind does? It wanders just like it does every other part of the day.

Neurolinguistic Programming

"Why is this so hard?" Kris asked me tearfully.

"Well," I said with a sigh, "there's a lot of things to overcome and unpack."

"Right, so like what's the point? I'm just tired of everything feeling so hard when it comes to my life," she said despairingly.

"I absolutely get that," I told her. "And I'm not just saying that to appease you. I'm saying it because that's how I used to feel also."

"You used to feel that way?" she asked me.

"Of course. All the time," I told her. "And sometimes, though it's rare now, that same thought will creep in. It's actually a belief."

"What do you mean?" she asked.

"I mean when I used to say, 'of course this would happen to me' or 'why is everything so hard,' I was expressing a belief I had about the world," I told her. "So when I would say, 'why is this so hard,' I was expressing the belief that life is hard. And hard is bad and obviously conspiring for my ultimate demise."

"I never thought about it like that," she said.

"Language is incredibly powerful," I explained. "Language affects everything. It affects how we show up. How we experience something. How we express things to our kids. Language keeps you stuck or moves you forward. Language can inspire and encourage or tear down and destroy. It's also a powerful indicator of what's happening internally. I'll let you in on a little secret. When my clients talk to me, I listen to not just what they say, but *how* they say it. It gives me insight into their beliefs."

"Interesting," she said.

"So someone may tell me that life is great and their marriage is great, but when something challenging comes along, I'm able to see whether their words match up to their beliefs," I explain.

"So what does my belief that life is hard say about me then?" she asked.

I smiled and said, "It could mean several things, but since I know your background and why you sought my help, I would say it means that you believe you're not worthy of good things, so of course life is hard."

"Why would I believe that though?" she asked. "I think I'm worthy of good things. I want good things."

"Absolutely," I began. "But that's the conscious brain talking. That's not the conditioned, collective unconscious mind talking. That's why those challenging moments are so insightful—they give us a peek into the unconscious mind and that's what runs the show about 95% of the time. You see, we only believe something because it serves us."

Kris pulled back a little and said, "How does believing I'm not deserving of good things serve me? That doesn't make sense."

"You're right," I stated. "It doesn't. This is what's called a secondary gain. What happens when you believe that you're not deserving of good things or really any other limiting belief? How do you show up?"

Kris considered my question. "Well, I guess...I really don't show up. I feel like I'm always kind of bracing myself for impact. For the other shoe to drop. So I am probably more resistant to opportunities and experiences because of that."

THIS IS A SECONDARY GAIN. And you have that same experience Kris did, just different details, limited by your own beliefs. I want you to consider what you've gained by not showing up for sex enthusiastically, by not loving your body or expecting and accepting pleasure. It feels counterintuitive to think that you wouldn't want these things, but that's exactly why it's been so hard to get different results than you've been getting. Because when you try and change a behavior, you get short-term results. You have to change the belief to get the true transformation.

I want you to get excited about releasing these limiting beliefs (let it go, let it go...). Giving them up and resist those voices telling you that you can't. We are here to claim our sacred sexual energy and harness it because it is ours to enjoy and explore. And as we've seen, limiting beliefs just get in the way of that. They keep us stuck. They keep us small and they rob us of the pleasures of life.

The Secret Sauce?

I'm sure you're wondering, ok so how do I get rid of these limiting beliefs that are keeping me miserable or unhappy? In short, there is no one-size-fits-all approach. And that is the beauty of the healing journey. There is no magic pill or secret sauce. So far, I've touched on several options, and I'll highlight two more for which I've been trained.

Many people have found great success with eye movement desensitization and reprocessing (EMDR). This is a therapeutic method that involves bilateral stimulation of the brain (i.e., activating both sides of the brain at the same time). This is done by tapping both knees or both shoulders or following a beeping horizontal light or the clinician's finger that moves side to side. The trauma or experience is slowly rewired and the intensity of the event dissipates so it's no longer triggering.

Most people find success with overcoming a fear or trauma in approximately 8 to 12 sessions. However, there has been some research showing that the efficacy of EMDR declines over time. Essentially, just because you rewire one trauma from your past doesn't mean that subsequent events can't impact your wellbeing. You still have to do the work to preserve your mental health.

One critical area of our bodies that is often overlooked when it comes to healing is our nervous system. Recalibrating your nervous system is really the foundation of any of the work you do. If we don't feel safe in our bodies (both at the conscious and unconscious level), then all the talk therapy in the world won't matter. Studies repeatedly show that children who come from homes where there is violence, poverty, and food insecurity have a much harder time learning in school. Why? Because they're in a state of hypervigilance and survival mode, so learning their time-tables isn't registered as a priority. When we feel safe in our environment, we flourish. When we feel safe in our body, we are open to transformation.

ALL THE TECHNIQUES and approaches discussed in this chapter require a guide. Can you do a lot of this work on your own? Sure. But you're going to spend a lot of time, money, and energy trudging this path alone. I cannot emphasize how important it is to work with a professional, whether that's a therapist or coach, mentor, or spiritual advisor. Finding a professional is a lot like dating. Just because you go to one appointment and don't have a great experience doesn't mean that all therapists are bad, just like all dates aren't bad. Be gracious to yourself as you navigate the search for someone you can trust, someone who is qualified to help you heal. But the healing is ultimately up to you. You are not broken, so they can't fix you. They can, however, show you the path and encourage you along the way.

Toolbox:

- How do I feel about the mind being multiple (having parts) versus just being one?

- What is a limiting belief I have? What is the secondary gain I get from having that belief?
- Do I feel safe in my body? When was the last time I felt safe in my body?
- What is preventing me from working with a professional to help me on my healing journey?

10

TOOLS TO TRANSFORM

"That all sounds great, Courtney, what you're saying," my friend told me. "But what does that actually look like in real life?"

"You mean you don't want to talk theory all day?" I asked her with a laugh.

"It makes sense," she continued. "I get why I don't want sex and why I'm not connected with my body. But what do I do about it? Where do I start?"

"Great questions," I told her.

THIS ACTUAL CONVERSATION is what led me to write this chapter. Because if I can't give you, the reader, tools to incorporate into your life, then I'm doing you a disservice. I've identified several practices to help you on your path. Find the ones that resonate with you. Be consistent. Diligent. Most of my clients experience a gradual transformation. Their flame doesn't turn into a bonfire overnight. It grows slowly and becomes more powerful the more attention and time they invest in it.

Also, be open to being uncomfortable. Growth never comes from a place of comfort. A caterpillar doesn't get to become a butterfly without first becoming a gross mess of goo. Some of these practices may be out of your comfort zone. That's ok! Try them anyways (unless, of course, they trigger a past trauma, in which case, please seek professional help). Most importantly, have fun. Make sex fun again! Or maybe for the first time. You can't mess these up. You can, however, develop them and make them work for you and your partner.

Sensual Living

In our modern times, we've become disconnected from the ways our bodies used to experience the world. We used to roam the earth barefoot, eat meals with our hands, and use our senses to navigate the world. For a variety of reasons, we've moved away from that. I believe that's cost us our connection to our senses. How can you rekindle that connection?

- Walk barefoot (bonus if it's outside in the grass or dirt).
- Eat your food with your hands instead of utensils (yes, it will be messier than usual; that's the point).
- Be aware of synthetic fragrances (candles, perfumes, and hair products); opt for essential oils or essences instead.
- Chew your food for at least 30 bites. Savor the flavor. Focus on the texture and taste.
- Focus on your breath. How does it feel coming into your nostrils? Focus on the out breath. Do you notice the warmth of it?
- Listen to music that makes your whole body want to move (and then move it!). Close your eyes and hear

the words. Feel the rhythm. Allow yourself to sway or
shake or jump.

- Try not using your smartphone to navigate. Yes, you
will probably get lost, but you may also discover
something along the way.

All the techniques listed above are ways to come home to
your body, which is really about coming home to yourself. Our
bodies want to be acknowledged, seen, and valued. Sensual
living is one way to do just that.

Sensate Focus

Sensate focus therapy is a great tool to use at any point in your
relationship. You don't have to be experiencing dysfunction to
explore this therapy with your partner. When I was first starting
out as a sex therapist, I had a client named Jane. Jane came to
me because she was struggling with vaginismus, a condition
where the muscles of the vagina involuntarily spasm, making
penetration difficult or painful. She was newly married, frustrated, and unhappy.

"MY HUSBAND HAS BEEN SO patient. We didn't have sex before we
got married and now that we're married, we can't even enjoy it,"
she began. "I don't know what to do. What's wrong with me?"
she tearfully asked me.

I smiled and said, "First of all there's nothing wrong with
you. It probably feels that way. We're going to figure it out, and
I'm here to help you."

I encouraged Jane to see a pelvic floor physical therapist to
help with the physical symptoms. Jane was able to find one and
began using dilators, phallic-shaped instruments used to stretch

the vagina. I began to work with Jane and her husband. I used sensate focus therapy to help them switch from penetrative sex (which Jane found stressful and painful) to pleasure-based sex.

Sensate focus combines mindfulness (being present in your body and allowing distracting thoughts to float away), exposure therapy (exposing oneself to an adverse experience in a relaxing, safe, and positive environment), and sensate touch (intentionally touching the body while only thinking about the temperature, pressure, or texture). I would assign them homework in which they would take turns sensually touching each other's bodies but would avoid the genital or chest area. The sensual touching would progress to eventually include these areas. The goal was to progress to the point of penetrative intercourse, without the pressure of having to orgasm. Again, the focus was on increasing the safety and pleasure of sexual intimacy for both partners.

One of the things I love about this modality is the focus on the senses. Here are some ways to expand your senses in sexual encounters (you can also apply many of these to solo sex):

- Use a blindfold. This heightens your other senses.
- Focus on the taste of your partner. How do their skin, lips, and yes, genitals, taste? Is their skin rough or soft? How does their body feel on your tongue?
- Breathe in your partner's scent. Does your own scent change when you become turned on?
- Listen to their breathing pattern. Does it quicken right before climax?
- Hold your breath right before you orgasm. It will lengthen and intensify orgasm.
- Take in the beauty of their body with your eyes. Notice how your partner looks at you. See yourself as the sexual being that you are.

- Safely utilize props like feathers, creams, foods, or
  even flogs, that offer different pressures,
  temperatures, textures, and tastes.

Many of us have been conditioned to be detached from our sexual experiences. Meaning we're not used to incorporating all our senses. Some of these exercises may feel overwhelming at first. Tuning into our bodies allows us to be fully turned on.

Cutting Sexual Lines

"I can't stop thinking about my ex," Yasmeen told me. "We broke up like six months ago, but I keep thinking about him."

"And that's upsetting you?" I asked her.

"Yes. Especially when I have flashbacks of us being together sexually. We had a great sex life and I miss that," she said sadly.

"Are you ready to really let him go, or do you feel like that's what you *should* want?" I inquired.

Yasmeen sighed. "No, I think I'm ready," she said confidently. "I want to move on and feeling this connection to him is preventing that."

I smiled and said, "Great. Let's do it."

SOMETHING NOT OFTEN DISCUSSED, even in the wooey world, is the presence of sexual energetic lines. If you're new to energy work and you're struggling to buy into this, that's ok! You don't have to believe in them, but I would encourage you to at least understand the belief system behind them.

One reason I believe this isn't discussed is the potential backlash of shaming a woman's sexual choices. I've seen some people state that women should limit their sexual partners (i.e., not outside of a committed monogamous relationship) because of the "damage" multiple sexual partners can have on them.

I WOULD BE REMISS if I didn't point out that sex is one of the most powerful ways we can exchange energy with another person. That statement is often used to justify regulating a woman's sexual behavior. So please know, I'm not here to tell you how many people you can or can't have sex with. Only you can make that decision. My aim here is to educate you on how being in a sexual relationship can affect you energetically.

How do you know if you have a sexual line to someone? The best way to tell is if you think about them often. Say you hooked up with someone in college and you haven't thought about them in 20 years. You likely don't have a sexual line with them.

Now, say you were dating someone in high school, and from time to time you find yourself thinking about being with them. It's likely you do have a sexual line with them. If you've been sexually assaulted, and you haven't done any healing work around the assault (therapy, energy work, etc...), it's likely you still have a sexual line to your assailant. In that specific instance, I highly recommend you find a professional who can help you through that healing process.

Sexual lines, and lines of any kind, can be cut a variety of ways. Many times they are cut through talk therapy, rituals such as burning a letter you wrote to your ex, or guided visualization exercises. One of the best ways to cut a line is to set the intention from a place of love, not anger. If you're still angry at your ex, then that needs to be addressed in addition to the sexual line cutting.

. . .

LET'S go back to my session with Yasmeen.

"Ok, I'm going to guide you through an exercise that will help cut the line you still feel with your ex," I told her. "First, go ahead and get comfortable in your seat, and if it feels safe, close your eyes. Now I want you to think about all the awful things that happened in your relationship. Things that he did or said to you that really bothered you or hurt you. And I want you to feel those in your body." I paused before asking her, "Do you feel them?"

"I do," she said calmly.

"Great," I said. "Now I want you to tell me or show me where in your body you feel them."

Yasmeen pointed to her heart.

"Excellent," I reassured her. "So just sit with those feelings. It's normal to feel uncomfortable. Remember, you are safe here. You're in control here. Now I want you to imagine that you're holding a beautiful satin white ribbon in front of you, like it's dangling from your hand. And I want you to picture all those feelings going from your heart into that white ribbon, like they're beaming out of you and being absorbed by this satin white ribbon." I paused, giving her time to process. "As you are experiencing these hard feelings leaving your body, I want you to tell me when you feel that space in your heart, where the unpleasant sensations were, is gone."

Again, I waited.

"Ok. It feels like there's a hole now where those feelings used to be," she said.

"Great," I told her. "Now I want you to imagine that in your other hand is a shiny pair of golden scissors. I want you to take those scissors and cut the ribbon in half. Let me know when you do that."

She paused before saying, "Ok I did it."

"Wonderful," I said. "Now let's bring your attention back to that empty space in your heart. What emotions do you want to have in this part of your body?"

Yasmeen thought for a few moments and then said confidently, "Peace. I want to feel peaceful. Calm, like a still stream."

"That's great," I told her. "Imagine that still stream exudes peace and calm and fills that part of your heart. Really feel that peace throughout your entire body and trust that you are no longer connected to your ex in any way. Believe that you are free, Yasmeen. And when you are ready, when this feels complete to you, open your eyes."

CUTTING lines is a potent way to take our power back. If this guided visualization doesn't resonate with you, that's ok! The important part is that you *feel* the harbored emotions, do something that signifies a detachment, and conclude by "installing" the way you want to feel going forward.

Movement

Movement is one way our body communicates. I remember dancing around the house as a child for no reason. There was no music, but it was as if my body just *had* to express itself in this way. I can still picture myself extending my arms and kicking up my feet. Bending my back and twisting my hands. I don't remember when I stopped moving this way, but I do remember why. Someone I loved saw me moving like this and told me that what I was doing was weird. In that moment, I believed (at an unconscious level) that moving my body like that, expressing my emotions through movement, wasn't safe. It led to judgment and rejection. So I stopped because acceptance was more important (and essential to my survival).

I've since come back to movement, though not as boldly as I

would love to be. I still find myself restricted and hesitant to move my body freely. I still fear judgment. But when I find myself in those moments, where I'm afraid to sway or shake or spin, I try to honor that little girl who danced like no one was watching. And I do it anyway.

Yoga

Yoga is healing through movement. There are countless advantages to this ancient practice. Studies repeatedly show the benefits of intentional breathing, the power of postures, and strength through stretching. Yoga is one of the gentlest and yet most powerful ways to connect with our bodies.

As we've explored throughout this book, many of us are disconnected from our bodies. It may not feel safe to inhabit your own skin. That is a normal response to T/trauma. In order to understand who we are, we must reconvene with the body we inhabit.

The practice of yoga can be a peaceful knock on the door of our hearts, allowing us to connect back to our bodies, to come home to ourselves. I love the philosophy of yoga:

- Look inward.
- Listen to your body.
- Notice your breath.
- Be in the present.
- Be curious.
- Know there is no competition or finish line.

There are so many variations of this ancient practice, so if you've tried a Vinyasa class and didn't love it, consider one of the many other options. I am by no means a yogi, but I have recently connected with Kundalini yoga. Kundalini yoga is a form of yoga that involves singing, breathing exercises, chanting, and repeated poses. Its purpose is to activate one's Kundalini (shakti) energy, located at the base of your spine.

Practicing this daily has increased my creativity, grounded me, and cultivated a strong sense of peace. Even though some days feel jam-packed and I'm tempted to skip out on this, I notice a difference (and so does my family) when I don't make this practice a priority.

One of the first yoga classes I went to was when my dad was dying. My neighbor asked me to join her at the studio in our small town. I really didn't want to go, but I thought it would be a good workout. I found the class challenging, but I was not prepared for what happened during Shavasana (the part where you lay on your back at the end of class).

I don't remember what the instructor said, but I remember tears pouring down my cheeks. I was so sad about my dad, so heartbroken. I tried to fight the tears, but I couldn't. I kept thinking, I'm going to be the crazy lady who cries at the end of a yoga class. Who does that? But I couldn't stop the tears. I couldn't stop the pain that was ready to be released. Yoga was the medium that allowed my heart to hurt. To really feel. I wish I could go back and tell myself that's exactly what my body needed me to do. Instead, I will tell you this—our bodies will find a way to release. The more connected we are with this truth, the more we are in control of when and how that happens. Honor that.

Know that you can practice any form of yoga. There are countless poses and practices for any- and everything. But the intention is usually the same—show up for yourself. Find the strength within you. Trust yourself. Challenge yourself. Discover that the secrets you have been holding don't want to stay hidden. They want to be released.

Because we can't receive if we're still holding onto old pain. And that can feel incredibly scary, if protecting that pain is all we've known. But true strength requires vulnerability. We release so we can receive. We lean in, knowing that we will find discomfort. And in that discomfort, we take a deep breath, believing that we can do it because we are stronger than we realize.

Sacral Chakra Poses

Because my focus was on activating my sacral chakra, I wanted poses that targeted the nourishment of the energy in this area. Since the sacral chakra is right below the belly button, any type of hip opening pose will work. There were so many to choose from, but I tried to vary them in terms of muscles used and positioning. When you do practice, I would encourage you to

- pay attention to how you feel doing these poses.
- really focus on your breathing. Do you notice certain poses cause you to shorten your breath?
- identify any sensations that come up in your body. Is there tightness? A sense of "stuckness?" Does any pose make you feel lighter? Stronger? More vulnerable?
- sit with and allow any feelings that come up during your practice. Let them wash over you.
- process any feelings that emerge through journaling.

If you don't know how to do these poses, Google is an excellent way to see them in action.

- Sukhasana (Easy Pose)
- Phalakasana (Plank Pose)

- Malasana (Garland Pose)
- Setu Bandha Sarvangasana (Bridge Pose)

Yoga reminds us that our bodies are an experience, not just placeholders for our souls. These poses allow us to be fully present, fully alive, in a part of us that may not have felt safe. That we may have avoided out of fear or shame. I want you to know that your body, especially this part of your body where your sexuality and sensuality and creativity and passion live, is beautiful—so beautiful. I hope these poses allow you to feel more connected to this truth.

Affirmations

Affirmations can be an incredibly potent tool to cultivate change. They can increase your awareness and allow you to set powerful intentions. What you're saying matters, but really it's HOW you're feeling when you say it that's incredibly important.

"EVERY DAY, I look in the mirror and say, 'you're beautiful, Kari, and you deserve good things,'" my client said to me. "And yet, I still don't actually believe those things."

"Is that how you say them?" I asked her. "Without any tone or emotion? Almost begrudgingly?"

"I mean, yeah," she responded. "I guess. I just say them and move on with my day."

"Sort of like another thing you can check off your list?" I asked Kari.

"Pretty much," she said.

"Unfortunately, affirmations don't work like that," I told her. "You have to believe them in order for them to work. Your body doesn't speak cognitive language, like we're talking right now; it only understands through FEELING."

"But I don't believe that I'm beautiful," she said. "And apparently I don't really believe I'm deserving of good things either."

"That's ok. You'll get there," I reassured her. "Here's what I want you to do. I want you to imagine, let's just pretend for a moment, that you actually DO believe that you're beautiful. Can you imagine that with me for just 30 seconds?"

Kari considered my question and said, "I mean sure, I guess I could."

"Ok, great," I told her. "Close your eyes. It probably would be helpful for you to avoid looking in the mirror while you're doing these affirmations. That can be a next step, but for now, if you feel comfortable, let's stick with just turning the focus inward by closing your eyes."

I waited for Kari to close her eyes and settle into her body.

"Now, I want you to imagine, remember, this is only for 30 seconds, that you actually DO feel beautiful," I instructed her. "You see yourself as beautiful. What does that FEEL like in your body?"

Kari's brow unfurrowed a bit and her breathing began to slow. Her shoulders relaxed and the biggest smile I had ever seen from her slowly emerged. She held this for about 10 seconds and then said, "I can't do this. This feels dumb." Defeated, her shoulders slumped and she dropped her head.

"Have you ever been to a scary movie?" I asked her.

Kari made a face, "Um, no. They're terrifying. Why would I subject myself to that?"

"But you know it's just pretend, right?" I said.

"Yeah, but my body doesn't know that," she stated.

And that's when it clicked. I smiled as I saw it all coming together for her.

She sat back in her chair, running her fingers through her hair and sighed. "Yep, ok, point made," she said.

"I don't know what you're talking about," I said playfully.

We sat in silence for a little while as she processed her realization. I broke the silence, "We have to get our bodies on board if we really want to change. Most people think that if we just tell our brains something, it will have what's called a 'top-down' effect, meaning that the body will get in line if we just tell our minds what to do. It doesn't work like that. Eighty percent of what we experience is processed from the bottom-up, meaning it goes through our body first. Only 20% goes through our brain first."

"So that's why these affirmations aren't working? My body doesn't believe it?" Kari asked me.

"I would say your body isn't *experiencing* your belief," I said. "Scary movies are exciting, well, for those who enjoy that sense of terror, because the body believes it's in those situations. It can't distinguish real from imaginary. It can only feel and sense. Our brains interpret those sensations and then make meaning out of it."

"But I don't believe that I'm beautiful, so how can I feel it?" Kari asked me.

"Sometimes we have to fake it till we make it. Sometimes we must recognize that this may not feel true right *now*, and that's ok. But we can want it to feel true, so we're going to focus on that. I like to think of this process like trying on clothes. I call it the Feelings Fitting Room. Do you remember trying clothes on in a store instead of just ordering them online?"

Kari laughed, "Yes, of course."

"Great," I said. "We're going to do just that, but with feelings. So first thing, identify how you want to feel. Let's say you want to feel confident. What thought would you need to think in order to feel confident?"

"For me, it would be something about being great at my job," she said.

"Ok, so something simple like 'I'm great at my job,'" I said.

She nodded her head, "yes."

"Now I want you to close your eyes," I told her. "And I want you to think that thought that you just identified, 'I'm great at my job,' and I want you to feel that confidence build inside you."

I watched Kari as she seemed to summon that thought and noticed a determined but confident look come across her face. I smiled and said, "That's it! You're doing it. Hold that feeling for 20 more seconds. Really *feel* that confidence."

After 20 seconds, I said to Kari, "Time's up." She slowly opened her eyes. I smiled, admiring her courage, and said, "That is how an affirmation should feel. Every time. That is how they work."

She nodded her head and said, "Ok. I get it now."

AFFIRMATIONS ARE one of the most misused tools. Hopefully reading about Kari's experience showed you how important it is to feel what it is you want to believe. Remember, it's not about going from believing something 50% to 100%. It's about going from 50 to 55. Then 55 to 60. It's moving the needle just a little, slowly, and steadily.

Eventually, in combination with the other work that contributes to cultivating your sacred sexual energy, these affirmations will get you from a place of disconnection and dissatisfaction to a place of love and acceptance. This will not happen overnight. Like everything else, change is the result of intentional daily practice.

Power of Sleep

One of my favorite times to do affirmations is right before bed because sleep is one of the BEST times to change your brain. In fact, research shows that sleep, specifically the state in which we dream, plays a significant role in regulating mood.

While the conscious mind is shut off, the subconscious mind is hard at work processing the day's events and communicating to us through dreams. We all dream, even if we don't remember them. Dreams provide an excellent opportunity to connect with your subconscious, which is where your limiting beliefs ultimately lie.

There are numerous ways to make this connection, but one method is through lucid dreaming. Lucid dreaming happens when the person consciously realizes they are asleep, but they do not wake up from their dream. Lucid dreaming allows you to actively participate in story lines that are created by your subconscious mind, kind of like directing a movie in your sleep. Dreams allow seemingly unrelated memories to make new connections, meaning that in our dream state, our conscious (judgmental) mind is offline. Nothing is preventing us from processing and experiencing.

Lucid dreaming takes this a step further and gives us control over this process. Because dreams repeat, re-fuse, and amalgamate old memories and information, they prompt what our conscious mind will notice and focus on as we go about our day. Individuals who practice lucid dreaming have been shown to have lower levels of anxiety and more creativity and are better problem solvers.

A simple way to prepare your brain for lucid dreaming is by repeatedly thinking right before you fall asleep, "I'm good at remembering my dreams. I'm good at lucid dreaming." You can also utilize other affirmations right before you fall asleep and those are what your brain will focus on as you sleep. Using a dream diary is also helpful. This allows you to recall what happened in your dreams (lucid or not) and process them when you're awake. Dream diaries can also serve as a way to track patterns of the types of dreams you're having, which may provide insight into messages your subconscious mind is trying to communicate.

Regulating Your Nervous System

As I briefly discussed in the last chapter, recalibrating your nervous system is really the foundation for any of the work you do. The more regulated your nervous system is, the more easily you are able to implement and integrate the various techniques into your daily life. Experiences become traumatic because they overwhelm our nervous system (and our emotions), which then puts us in a dysregulated state.

In order to be more present in our bodies, we need our nervous system regulated. The state you are in (fight, flight, freeze, or fawn) will determine the techniques you use. So if you're in a freeze state (the dorsal vagal state), taking long deep breaths actually won't be helpful. You need something to energize you from that freeze state (e.g., more rapid breathing).

I've identified some exercises that can help you regulate your nervous system (just be mindful of the fight, flight, freeze, or fawn state you're in). Pay attention to how these techniques feel during and after you complete them:

- Take long, deep breaths to bring down your heart rate, lower cortisol levels, and soothe your mind and body (if you're in a fight or flight state). Put one hand on your belly and one hand on your heart. Breathe in through your nose and out slowly through your nose

or mouth, with each inhalation and exhalation
lasting at least 5 seconds.

- Immerse yourself in cold water by taking an ice bath
  or cold shower or even by splashing cold water on
  your face to stimulate the vagus nerve and "shock"
  the system into a more regulated state.
- Stimulate the throat chakra through singing or
  humming.
- Go for a silent walk in nature (also known as forest
  bathing) or near bodies of water (without music or
  other distractions)
- Shake your body (if you're in a fight or flight state)
- Engage in an activity that is both social and physical
  (e.g., team sports or a spin class) to move to a calmer
  state.
- Gently tap your arms and legs with a closed palm (if
  you're in a freeze state)

These techniques are meant to move you from an immobilized, survival response to one that is regulated, restored, and rooted in resilience. Sometimes it isn't easy to identify which state your nervous system is in. The more you connect with your body, the easier it is to identify which state you're in and which technique is most effective for you in that dysregulated state.

Forgiveness

I've talked with my clients about forgiveness countless times over the years. I've worked with individuals whose lives were shattered by abuse and betrayal. I've worked with couples whose relationships were plagued by mistrust and heartbreak. Time and time again, I come back to the truth that the only way forward is through forgiveness.

And that is easy to say when you don't have anything invested in that scenario. When you're on the outside looking in, telling someone to just, "let it go." To forgive and move forward.

I recently found myself in a position where I needed to practice what I had preached for so long. And let me tell you, it was much harder to offer grace and forgiveness to someone than I anticipated. So I won't tell you to just forgive and forget and move right along! But I will encourage you to consider the cost of not forgiving. Because when we harbor anger towards someone, we slowly poison ourselves. We are the ones that suffer, not them.

Resentment is one hell of an effective shield. It keeps out the bad. It doesn't let the pain in. The problem is that it also keeps out the good. The love. The joy. And it also keeps us from growing. Prevents our hearts from expanding.

One of my favorite ways to offer forgiveness is through a traditional Hawaiian forgiveness ritual called *Ho'oponopono*, which roughly translates to "make things right" or "move things back into balance." It's simple and yet incredibly profound. I've practiced this twice in the last year and have felt such freedom from it. When you decide you are ready to forgive, when you are ready to release your past and the behaviors of others, consider this ritual.

Find a quiet place to sit. Close your eyes and repeat this mantra: *"I'm sorry, Please forgive me, Thank you, I love you."* That's it. You may need to repeat it many times. You may only need to say it once. For some, this is a gradual process. It is totally fine if this does not feel easy-peasy. It doesn't mean you're doing anything "wrong." Letting go can feel very scary and our brains don't like scary.

These words, *"I'm sorry, Please forgive me, Thank you, I love you,"* are meant to cultivate a sense of self love and inner peace inside you. It's critical to know that this is not about excusing what the person did. It's not about absolving them from their transgressions. It's about you taking your power back through an act of love. An act that they probably don't deserve but you sure as hell do.

Healing

I used to believe that healing followed a linear path. In graduate school, I was trained in the widely popular cognitive behavioral therapy modality. In its simplest form, you guide your client to a better life by changing the way they think, which changes the way they feel, which changes the way they act. Having trouble getting to Point C? Change your Points A and B. Easy-peasy.

But what I have found in working with clients for so many years and in my own personal journey is that healing takes anything but a straight path. Most of the time it looks like a preschooler trying to draw you a picture. There are lines everywhere and you can't really figure out where they started or what the final product is. But you know that there's movement because you can't help but see those thick impressions on that paper. All over that page.

That is the healing journey. And honestly, all these tips and tricks won't do you any good if you're not in the healing arena. On the field, in the game, suited up and ready to go. And man, is that scary. Because we want to believe that we can just think ourselves into a better life. Into more sex or more creativity or whatever. Unfortunately, it's just not that simple. And anyone who tells you it is, isn't seeing the big picture or being totally transparent.

Transformation, true change, can't happen independently from healing. It's a critical part of the recipe. One that many of us like to pretend we don't need. But just like that cake won't rise without a leavening agent, the changes we want, the ones that truly last, won't stick unless we're committed to healing. And we can only heal through love. The more we love, the more we heal, and the more we are healed, the more we are able to love.

But loving requires vulnerability. And vulnerability makes us susceptible to suffering. I believe those are the only two ways that transformation occurs—through love and suffering. They're the two sides of the transformation coin. Suffering is not a consequence, though it often feels like one. And love is not a reward. But it is the cure. Not in the one-and-done sense, where you pop a pill and move back on with your day.

No, love is the patient guide that accompanies us on our journey. That forever friend who reminds us, sometimes in a not so gentle way, that we are here. That we are held. And that we are capable of creating a life that we are worthy of.

These practices aren't just about getting you to have more sex. I mean, sure, maybe that's part of it. Sex is a tangible act of tuning into this creative channel. But maybe it's not. Here's what this work is all about. It's about loving yourself, honoring the sacred sexual energy inside of you, and believing that you can be liberated. To dream and desire big. To create. To laugh. To enjoy. To love. To breathe. To express your sovereignty by claiming what resides within you.

That flame that wants to burn bright and bring forth something more is inside you. May you honor that power within you and know that you are worthy of all that you desire.

Toolbox:

- Identify one tool discussed in this chapter and decide how you will incorporate that into your life.
- Is there anyone in my past or present who I need to forgive? What is preventing me from doing this?

- Imagine you're in the Feelings Fitting Room. What feeling do you want to try on? What thought do you need to think in order to feel that? Practice trying it on for 30 seconds and focus on how it feels in your body.
- Create a right-before-bedtime affirmation that programs your subconscious mind right before you fall asleep. Commit to doing it every night.

11

SEXPECTATIONS

"Honestly, I could go without sex, for like ever, maybe? I mean, at least for a few months," Sarai shared with me during our session.

"Why do you think that is," I asked her.

She seemed confused by the question, giving a small smirk. "Because it's just one more thing I have to do," she stated as she shook her head. "I'm tired," she continued. "It's really just another box to check at this point. Another reminder of how I'm failing as a wife..."

I asked her, "Was it always like this? Was there ever a time when you didn't feel like it was just another thing on your to-do list?"

She tilted her head to think for a minute, "Hmm, probably. But that feels so long ago. It feels like a lifetime ago. I don't even remember what it was like before kids and work and all these meetings. There's just so much pressure on me all the time. Sex is just one more thing, you know?"

I shook my head yes because I did know.

. . .

So MANY OF the women I talk to see sex as just one more thing. And not just one more thing you have to do, but one more thing you have to be engaged in. For many women, sex feels like a performance. They have to get dressed up (sexy lingerie), make sure they look good (Showered? Shaved? Smell good?) to put on a show. For other women, they've let most of this effort go, but still find themselves uninterested in any sexual acts.

When you see sex as another thing you must do or perform, it's going to drain your energy. And it's hard to become aroused when you're limping into bed every night from exhaustion. Mainstream media does not help with this matter. Shows and movies are filled with couples climaxing together and rolling over to fall asleep in each other's arms. That's not reality. If that's your experience, fantastic. But most of the individuals I work with struggle with being authentic in their sexual relationships (e.g., faking orgasms). Being our authentic selves, especially in our sexual relationships, is just not something we're taught. So please don't get discouraged if you have absolutely no idea how to do that.

I promise it's not as complicated as it sounds.

If you're starting to incorporate the things you've learned throughout this book, you're already starting to shift to a more authentic, a more connected, a more compassionate version of yourself. And that's the best kind of place to be, especially during intimate acts.

One way to tune into this is by assessing your goal for sex. Is it to just check a box? Meet your partner's sexual needs? Fulfill a duty? Is it driven by a sense of obligation or guilt? Women have sex for a multitude of reasons (one study noted over 200). Sadly, most of the time women agree that having sex has nothing to do with their own needs or desires. Rather, it's for their partner.

It's important to be honest with yourself here. Because when we're honest with ourselves, we choose to live authentically. We face our circumstances head on and decide how we want to feel about it. Taking responsibility can feel scary, but it's necessary to create a life that feels full of integrity. So please, be honest with yourself, and once you are, consider this—would you want to have sex with someone who was only doing it with you because they felt like they had to? (Crickets, crickets...). No! You wouldn't. So why would you assume that your partner would?

"But it's so much work!" Danae shared.

"Of course it is," I nodded in agreement.

She looked at me confused, like wait, you're not supposed to agree with me.

I continued, "It's work when you look at it like another job. Another task. Another performance. Another set of expectations you have to meet. And when you have a history of not meeting those expectations (in other words, orgasming when you're 'supposed to'), you avoid those situations because of how you feel in them."

"Yes! Exactly," she replied.

Here's what I told her.

If the goal of sex is to orgasm, then there's a pressure to perform. We don't want that. Sex is meant to be fun. Let me repeat that. Sex is meant to be fun. Unless you're getting paid to put on a show, which I assume you're not, then remind your inner critic—that part of you that believes you must orgasm or must have sex for a certain amount of time—that you appreciate it looking out for you. And then tell it that you're ready to change how you look at sex.

What if you changed the goal of sex from performance to pleasure? If the goal of sex is pleasure and connection, it removes the need to climax. Remember, pleasure is a gift. It's what keeps us connected to an experience. Pleasure allows us to demonstrate and receive affection and attention. Pleasure connects us with our senses. Pleasure opens up the possibilities of playfulness. A pleasured woman is a woman connected to her desires, which are directly linked to her purpose.

As you consider changing the lens through which you view sex, I want you to listen to any parts of you that are resistant to accepting that. Our brains like predictability. They like to know when something begins and ends. When there's a performance, there's a clear ending (in this case, orgasm or ejaculation). It's important to note that most of my clients go through a gradual transformation of the way they view sex. They must intentionally come back to their conditioning of sex as performance-based and choose to see it differently. This does not happen overnight for most women.

With this new outlook, when sex is a pleasurable experience and not a performance, there is no natural ending. And for the taskmaster typically running our brains, this can feel uncomfortable: "I don't have time to have sex for hours, Courtney. I have things to do!" I promise, I'm not going to tell you that you need to have sex for hours on end. I mean, unless you really want to; in that case, I will give you a wink, and say, "get it, girl."

THIS IS why having clear sexpectations, expectations around sex, is so, so important. Sexpectations lay the foundation for frequency, among other things, which is one of the issues couples argue about most. Have you ever asked your partner how often they want to have sex? I asked a client this once in a couple's session. "Lee, how many times a week do you think your spouse wants to have sex?" She laughed, "Um, every day if he could." Straight-faced, I asked, "Have you ever asked him that?" Her laughing stopped, "Uh, I don't think so. I just assumed that because it feels like he asks for it all the time." I smiled, "Ok, well, now's your chance to ask him."

We make up these stories in our head. We tell ourselves things that don't always serve us. And instead of challenging their validity, we accept them as truths. A lot of times this happens because talking about sex, about our desires and needs, makes us uncomfortable. Sex is a vulnerable act, even with the lights off. And our brains don't like vulnerable. It puts us at risk on all the levels, especially if you've been hurt or abused sexually in the past.

"I know this can feel uncomfortable, talking about sex," I told Gabby. I wanted to shift the focus back to her. Back to what she had control over, but had likely never considered. "How often would you like to have sex?"

She shrugged, "I don't know. I've never really thought about it."

I smiled, "That's ok! So that will be your homework. I want you to think about how often you would want to have sex, if it weren't based on performance. If it was just a time for you and your partner to connect and have fun. To give and receive pleasure. No agenda and no expectations."

She agreed, "Yeah, I can do that."

The next week, Gabby came back and shared, "I'm finding it's hard for me to even think about my partner sexually or about sex at all when there's a pile of dishes in the sink and the kids have soccer practice, and you know, life!"

I reassured her, "Absolutely. These are realities we have to work with." I asked her, "Do you find that you have sexpectations that apply outside the bedroom?"

She seemed unclear, "I don't know what you mean."

I responded, "What I see happen a lot is that we have these unwritten operating instructions, just like you would for a refrigerator or an iPhone, that indicate how we want our partners to operate. We expect them to serenade or woo us, help with the kids, do the dishes first, and THEN we'll show up for them in bed. Like, you did all these things for me, so now I'm ready to put out for you. You're welcome. Does that make sense?"

She nodded her head, "Oh, I see now. Hmm. Probably. I mean, I don't really think it's fair that he expects me to just be ready to get it on when he hasn't helped out around the house all day."

"Of course," I told her. "Have you told him that?"

She pursed her lips together and shook her head, "No."

THERE IS nothing wrong with having sexpectations. If you expect your partner to do x, y, or z before you're ready to get it on, TELL. THEM. THAT. Don't play games. Don't be passive aggressive: "Oh I see the dishes are still in the sink..." and then use that as a reason to withdraw sexually; instead, communicate. Communicate these sexpectations to your partner. I'm sure you've heard this before, but communication is key. It helps reduce resentment and it increases intimacy. Obviously *how* you communicate matters also. I'm a big fan of communicating respectfully and constructively.

Toolbox:

- When was the last time you laughed during sex? Or flirted during foreplay? Sex doesn't need to be serious. It's meant to be fun!

- Identify your sexpectations (frequency, prerequisites, etc.) and then communicate those to your partner.
- Create a recurring check-in (once a month or quarter) so you and your partner can discuss whether your sexual needs are being met (Does the frequency need to change? The environment?)

CONCLUSION: THE COLLECTIVE

Until I started doing the research for this book, I never really understood how pervasive and problematic the messaging was around women's bodies and our sexuality. Sure, I knew that there was a "problem." I mean who hasn't had body image issues or a low desire for sex?

What I failed to take into account was the millennia of malfeasance women have faced. The micro- and macromessaging that a woman's body is not her own and really just exists for the pleasure and convenience of others. I could go on and on, but we've covered a lot of this already. The bottom line is that our issues go deep—way deep.

But they're not just our issues. They're everyone's. Because what affects one (statistically significant) portion of the population matters. And for a long time, women have not been made to feel that we mattered. More so, we haven't believed that we've mattered.

So when it comes to something as seemingly silly as low interest in sex or pain during sex or hating our bodies, people haven't really paid attention. It's a woman's issue. And because women don't really matter, their issues sure as hell don't matter either. So we never get the attention we deserve. And I don't mean someone nicely listening to us pour out our hearts. I mean funding for research that focuses on the vagina, uterus, and clitoris. I mean policies that protect a woman's right to her own body. I mean clinicians trained to look at women and their experiences differently.

I hope and pray that this book helps women understand that not being interested in sex isn't just a personal problem. It's deeper than that. It's a problem that goes so far into the soil, like the roots of a tree. Because when we all start to realize how interconnected we are, we start to see our interactions, our communication, our behaviors, differently.

And that is how we truly begin to heal. Together. And together we can find freedom. To live. To love. To decide for ourselves what feels nourishing and life-giving and what is not worthy of our time and attention. Because that is what I want for you. To see and believe that you are worthy of wonderfully pleasurable things. You always have been, sister. May you find them and may they bring you unspeakable joy.

ACKNOWLEDGMENTS

I finished this book a week before my grandma died. She loved to edit my essays in high school and college. I hated that red pen of hers. But I wouldn't be here if it weren't for her constant grammatical corrections and the belief that my words could make a difference in the lives of others. Thank you, Grams.

To my husband, Nathan. Who has seen me grow more than anyone. Thank you for believing in me and this crazy dream of writing a book. I love you.

To my kids. Addison, Avery, and Asher. Someday you will read these words and understand why I do the work I do. I hope I make you proud. Thank you for encouraging me to finish this book when I felt like giving up.

To my mom and dad. You have always believed in me. I am forever grateful for your love and support.

To my sister. My best friend and fellow purity culture survivor. Who knows where I'd be without you.

To my book coach, Emily. You helped bring this vision forward. Your encouragement, guidance, and support is something I will always be grateful for. This book is what it is because of you.

To my beta readers. Chelsea, Kelsey, Sarah, Brooke, and Jamie. Your comments and suggestions were so appreciated and helped shape the finality of this book. Thank you.

To my clients. Your stories. Your vulnerability. Your courage. I hope you see that you are not alone in your struggles.

To my friends. Who asked me how my book was coming. Who believed in me enough to care.

To my photographer and hair stylist. Liz, thank you for bringing out my beauty and asking how you can support this book.

To my friend and mentor. Meg, you conveyed where I needed to begin and helped start me on this path. Thank you.

To that little girl. Who sat down countless times at her childhood desk. Desperate to write something that mattered. We did it. Thank you for not giving up.

ABOUT THE AUTHOR

Born and raised in coffee country (looking at you, Seattle), Courtney Boyer is passionate about helping others. After marrying her college sweetheart in 2005, she began her career in sexuality education and counseling. Courtney is the founder of Courtney Boyer Coaching, a speaker, author, mother of three, and running enthusiast. She has never strayed from her coffee roots and enjoys meeting new people over a steaming cup of joe (or glass of red wine). Courtney and her family live abroad and enjoy traveling.

Printed in Great Britain
by Amazon

41542219R00099